Workbook to Accompany

Surgical Technology: Principles and Practice

5th Edition

Prepared by
Janet Milligan, RN, CNOR
Associate Professor for Surgical Technology
College of Southern Idaho
Twin Falls, Idaho

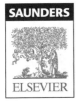

SAUNDERS

ELSEVIER

D1380088

SAUNDERS
ELSEVIER

3251 Riverport Lane
Maryland Heights, Missouri 63043

WORKBOOK TO ACCOMPANY SURGICAL TECHNOLOGY: ISBN 978-1-4160-6192-2
PRINCIPLES AND PRACTICE
Copyright © 2010, 2005 by Saunders, an imprint of Elsevier Inc.

Notice

ISBN 978-1-4160-6192-2

Publishing Director: Andrew Allen
Acquisitions Editor: Jennifer Janson
Associate Developmental Editor: Kelly Brinkman
Publishing Services Manager: Julie Eddy
Project Manager: Rich Barber

Working together to grow
libraries in developing countries

www.elsevier.com | www.bookaid.org | www.sabre.org

ELSEVIER   BOOK AID   Sabre Foundation
            International

Printed in the United States

Last digit is the print number: 9 8 7 6 5 4 3 2 1

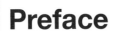

Preface

The goal of this workbook is to help students apply and master key concepts and skills presented in *Surgical Technology: Principles and Practice, 5th edition*. The exercises in this workbook will reinforce comprehension of material from the textbook.

The following exercises will provide a sufficient review of concepts and will allow the student to apply the concepts from the text:

- Each chapter begins with a *key term* review. A list of important terms in the corresponding book chapter is provided to test student comprehension of main concepts.
- **Short Answer** response questions apply knowledge learned from the text to a variety of situations.
- A variety of question formats test knowledge of concepts in the book, including **matching**, **true/false**, and **multiple choice**.
- **Labeling** exercises reinforce important anatomy concepts a surgical technologist should be familiar with.
- **Case Studies** provide the practical skills of being a surgical technologist. Patient scenarios allow students to be familiar with real-life situations that will prepare them for the job.
- **Internet Exercises** guide students in finding answers to current, important patient care and health issues facing the medical community today.

Best wishes as you begin your journey to become a surgical technologist!

Contents

1 The Surgical Technologist

Student's Name _____

KEY TERMS

Write the definition for each term.

1. ACS _____

2. Allied health profession _____

3. AST _____

4. Certification _____

5. Circulator _____

6. Continuing education _____

7. CST-CFA _____

8. Delegation _____

9. Dependent tasks _____

10. Independent tasks _____

11. Licensure _____

12. National Board of Surgical Technology and Surgical Assisting (NBSTSA) _____

_____

13. National Center for Competency Testing (NCCT) _____

_____

14. Nonsterile team members _____

15. Proprietary school _____

16. Surgical conscience _____

SHORT ANSWERS

Provide a short answer for each question or statement.

17. What are the differences between the titles TS-C and CST and ORT? _____

_____

_____

18. What is an ARC/STSA, and what is the job of the ARC/STSA?

_____

_____

19. What are the educational options for a student who would be educated in surgical technology? _____

_____

_____

20. Why is it important for a practicing surgical technologist to engage in continued education? _____

_____

_____

21. Name three areas of potential employment for a graduate surgical technologist.

_____

_____

22. What is the role of the surgical educator?

_____

_____

23. What is the difference between a surgical educator and a surgical clinical preceptor?

_____

_____

24. What is the difference between empathy and sympathy?

_____

_____

25. What do you think is the difference between having good organizational skills and being able to prioritize tasks?

_____

_____

26. Why does the AST organization need or want to work on legislative actions?

_____

_____

27. What are the additional educational requirements for a surgical technologist to become a surgical first assistant?

_____

_____

28. Name three places where a graduate surgical technologist might find employment.

_____

_____

MATCHING I

Match each term with the correct definition.

29. _____ Accreditation Review Council on Education in Surgical Technology and Surgical Assisting

30. _____ Association of periOperative Registered Nurses

31. _____ Professional association for surgical technologists

32. _____ Nonprofit organization that provides certification examination for surgical technologists trained in the military

33. _____ Commission that accredits allied health programs

a. ARC/STSA

b. CAAHEP

c. AST

d. AORN

e. NCCT

MATCHING II

Match each term with the correct definition.

34. _____ Requires supervision

35. _____ May be done by a surgical technologist without direction

36. _____ Transfer of responsibility for an activity from one person to another

37. _____ A task such as preparing surgical equipment

38. _____ A task such as retracting tissues during a procedure

39. _____ A task such as performing a surgical hand scrub

40. _____ A task such as maintaining the surgical field

41. _____ A task such as preparing medications for the surgeon

a. Independent task

b. Delegation

c. Dependent task

Indicate whether the statement is true or false.

42. Allied health professionals have a distinct expertise that is both humanistic and technical.

    _____ True   _____ False

43. National certification for surgical technology can be obtained in several ways. One way is through the NBSTSA, and another other way is through the NCCT.

    _____ True   _____ False

44. ORT was a career developed by the U.S. Army when a need arose during World War II.

    _____ True   _____ False

45. The surgical technologist educator must be a registered nurse.

    _____ True   _____ False

46. An example of a nonsterile person in the operating room is the circulator.

    _____ True   _____ False

47. Once a surgical technologist begins working, the qualities of empathy and caring can be enhanced through personal growth or lost through job stress.

    _____ True   _____ False

48. The U.S. military continues to educate surgical technologists today.

    _____ True   _____ False

49. The AST only provides its members opportunities for attending national conferences.

    _____ True   _____ False

50. National certification is always achieved by surgical technology students before they graduate from an accredited program of study.

    _____ True   _____ False

51. One of the tasks the organization called the AST performs is to participate in state and national legislative activities.

    _____ True   _____ False

52. No formal code of ethics has been established for the career of surgical technology.

    _____ True   _____ False

4

53. The surgical technologist knows how to clean and sterilize instruments and can troubleshoot problems with all types of equipment.

_____ True   _____ False

54. Serving as surgical technology clinical preceptor does not require patience and a willingness to share knowledge and experience.

_____ True   _____ False

55. Emotional maturity is the inability to control strong feelings and vent them appropriately in a constructive manner.

_____ True   _____ False

MULTIPLE CHOICE

Choose the most correct answer for each question or statement.

56. Which of the following is NOT considered a health career?
    a. Emergency medical technologists
    b. Nuclear medicine technicians
    c. Surgical technologists
    d. Registered nurses

57. In the past two decades, _____ has caused an enormous increase in the number and education of allied health professionals.
    a. Increased pay for technologists
    b. An increase in the number of hospitals needing surgical technologists
    c. An increase in technology
    d. An increase in the number of high school graduates

58. AORN first began formally training surgical technologists, using the organization's published manual, in _____.
    a. 1945
    b. 1950
    c. 1967
    d. 1970

59. Which of the following organizations is considered the professional organization for surgical technologists?
    a. NBSTSA
    b. AORN
    c. LCC-ST
    d. AST

60. Which of the following organizations sets the standards and guidelines for operating rooms?
    a. NBSTSA
    b. AORN
    c. LCC-ST
    d. AST

61. Which of the following organizations is responsible for overseeing program accreditation for the Commission on Accreditation of Allied Health Education Programs?
    a. AST
    b. ARC/STSA
    c. LCC-ST
    d. AORN

62. Surgical technology (as a profession) is a(an) _____ profession.
    a. Regulated
    b. Unregulated
    c. Transitional
    d. Registered

63. In surgical technology, national certification is _____.
    a. Mandated by each state
    b. Voluntary
    c. Licensed
    d. Regulated by the state Board of Nursing

64. _____ provide(s) an opportunity for professionals to improve their knowledge and competency throughout a career.
    a. Certification
    b. Continuing education
    c. Work experience
    d. Licensure and state registration

65. Which of the following is NOT one of the goals of the surgical technology clinical ladder?
    a. Improving patient care
    b. Increasing revenue for the hospital or surgery center
    c. Promoting accountability
    d. Encouraging employer recognition

66. If you graduated from a surgical technology program and took a job in materials management or CSP, which of the following would be included in your job description?
    a. Sterilization and disinfection
    b. Maintenance of the sterile surgical field
    c. Assisting with the procedure
    d. Mopping the floor and making the OR table

67. Which of the following is NOT one of the five specific domains of surgical technology?
    a. Assisting as part of the surgical team
    b. Preparing and handling the surgical equipment and tools
    c. Leadership, management, and education
    d. Providing postoperative patient care

68. Which of the following are considered positive or desirable attributes for a successful surgical technologist? (Select all that apply.)
    a. Honest
    b. Empathetic
    c. Uncooperative interpersonal relationships
    d. Caring

69. Which of the following best defines the characteristics of empathy?
    a. The ability to comprehend another person's feelings
    b. Feeling sorry for another person
    c. A singular emotional reaction to another persons, condition
    d. Recognition that the other person has very little worth

70. In the profession of surgical technology, manual dexterity is _____.
    a. Not needed because the instruments are assembled in central sterile processing
    b. Required so that the surgical technologist might work quickly and deftly
    c. Defined as keeping the instruments organized
    d. Required to keep the surgical technologist focused

MATCHING III

Match each role of the surgical technologist with the correct category of the associated duties.

71. _____ Surgical technologist who is "scrubbed"

72. _____ Surgical technologist who is NOT considered sterile

73. _____ Surgical technologist who wears a gown and gloves

74. _____ Surgical technologist who may assist in the circulating duties

a. Sterile duties

b. Nonsterile duties

Case Study 1

Read the following case study and answer the questions based on your knowledge of the scope of practice for a surgical technologist.

You are a surgical technologist who has been hired as a new graduate in the local surgery center. You have worked there for about a month, and a seasoned Certified Surgical Technologist is still acting as your preceptor. You have been assigned to work with Dr. Smith, who will be performing an open inguinal hernia procedure. You have never worked with this surgeon before. Once the procedure begins, the surgeon asks you to administer the local anesthetic. You know that as a surgical technologist, you are not allowed to administer medications.

75. Has the surgeon just delegated to you the task of administering the local anesthetic?

76. Is administration of a local anesthetic within your scope of practice?

77. Would the situation be different if you had been passing the instruments and your preceptor had been assisting?

78. What could you do in this situation?

Read the following case study and answer the questions based on your knowledge of certification options for a surgical technologist.

You have worked in an operating room for the past 15 years. Your hospital recently merged with another local hospital. The new combined hospital has asked that all surgical technologists become certified within the next 12 months. You were trained on the job; you did not graduate from an accredited program and are not eligible to take the exam through the NBSTSA.

79. Can you become certified?

80. What are your other options for certification?

81. What are the requirements for the alternate certification process?

82. If you were to become certified with one of the options you listed for question 80, do you have to take a national exam?

83. What would your title be if you became certified with the organization you listed?

84. If you are not certified with the NBSTSA, can you join the Association of Surgical Technologists as a professional organization?

INTERNET EXERCISES

Internet Exercise 1

Go online to the AST Web site to research your future career in surgical technology. Using the Web site, answer the following questions.

85. What is the average pay for a surgical technologist nationally?

86. What is the average pay for a surgical technologist in the state where you live?

87. Can you find your surgical technology program on the Web site listed under accredited programs?

88. Who is the accrediting body for your school's program?

89. Are student services listed on the Web site? If so, what are they? If not, what services do you think you would like to find?

90. Can you find any surgical technology scholarships offered on the Web page? If so, what are they?

91. Where (and when) is the AST national convention being held?

Internet Exercise 2

Go online to NBSTSA at www.lcc-st.org. Search the site for information about the certifying examination and answer the following questions.

92. Can you find any free materials that the NBSTSA could send you or that you could download to help you study for the certifying exam?

93. Is there a link on the NBSTSA Web page to other surgical professional organizations?

94. What process must you follow to apply for and take the examination?

95. While searching the site, what information did you find that told you the cost of the examination? Were any services or reduction in cost available for students?

96. Does any information on the site suggest why a graduate would like to take a national exam?

Internet Exercise 3

Using your favorite search engine, go online and search for study guides for the surgical technology certifying exam. Use the site or sites to answer the following questions.

97. Where did you find books to purchase?

98. Did you find more than one study guide? If so, what are the titles?

99. How much did they cost?

2 The Patient in Surgery

Student's Name _____

KEY TERMS

Write the definition for each term.

1. Body image _____
2. Critical thinking _____
3. Cultural competence _____
4. Elimination _____
5. Maslow's hierarchy _____
6. Mobility _____
7. Nutrition: _____
8. Outcome-oriented care _____
9. Patient-centered care _____
10. Physiological _____
11. Reflection _____
12. Regression _____
13. Relational _____
14. Respiration _____
15. Self-actualization _____
16. Therapeutic communication _____
17. Thermoregulation _____
18. Ventilation _____

SHORT ANSWERS

Provide a short answer for each question or statement.

19. What is the difference between patient-centered care and outcome-oriented patient care?

_____

_____

20. Patient _____ care would be more likely to use the information found by making a Maslow chart.

21. Why would a patient feel a loss of security if he or she were about to undergo a surgical procedure?

_____

_____

22. How are self-image and body image related?

_____

_____

23. Being in love and having a positive, happy relationship are part of the _____ domain of Maslow's hierarchy of needs.

24. Therapeutic responses include _____.

25. Your special population patient, who is _____ (age), is most at risk for skin tears or injury.

26. The normal aging process does not include _____.

27. The needs of a person are summarized by a theory called _____.

28. Cultural competence includes respect and acknowledgment of _____.

29. Violation of a patient's _____ can result in serious sanctions, including termination of employment.

MATCHING

Match each of the following terms, which deal with Maslow's triangular hierarchy, with the correct definition.

30. _____ Sleep
31. _____ Temperature
32. _____ Mobility
33. _____ Safety
34. _____ Security
35. _____ Belonging
36. _____ Altered body image
37. _____ Achieving personal goals
38. _____ Elimination
39. _____ Respiration
40. _____ Love
41. _____ Nutrition

a. Physiological
b. Protection
c. Relational
d. Self-actualization

Indicate whether the statement is true or false.

42. Senile dementia is a disease state.

_____ True   _____ False

43. The surgical technologist's role is focused on safety, advocacy, and psychosocial support.

_____ True   _____ False

44. In patient-centered care, the surgical team bases assessment, planning, and intervention on the unique needs of the individual patient.

_____ True   _____ False

45. Many patients approach surgery with anxiety and fear.

_____ True   _____ False

46. The patient feels greater security when team members do not discuss with them their upcoming procedure or the potential outcomes of the procedure.

_____ True   _____ False

47. Therapeutic communication is goal oriented.

_____ True   _____ False

48. Knowledge of our own attitudes helps clarify and prepare our response to the patient.

_____ True   _____ False

49. It is impossible for professionals to prevent their own beliefs from interfering with patient care or from allowing them to judge another.

_____ True   _____ False

50. Reassurance and open acknowledgment of the patient's fears are good methods of communicating empathy.

_____ True   _____ False

51. Many patients are afraid of *anesthesia awareness,* which is the state of being awake or aware of the procedure being performed.

_____ True   _____ False

52. Appropriate therapeutic communication requires a nonjudgmental and supportive attitude.

_____ True   _____ False

53. Spirituality is not necessarily the same as religion, although they often are expressed as one entity.

_____ True   _____ False

54. Health care professionals have an ethical responsibility to honor and respect the beliefs of patients of different cultures, just as they would want their own beliefs to be honored in a different culture.

_____ True   _____ False

55. Patients who are considered immunocompromised are at greatest risk for nosocomial infections.

_____ True   _____ False

56. Touch is NOT an important part of therapeutic communication.

_____ True   _____ False

MULTIPLE CHOICE

Choose the most correct answer for each question or statement.

57. Which of the following special populations would be at greatest risk for impaired wound healing?
   a. Infants
   b. Elderly
   c. Adolescents
   d. Diabetic patients

58. A _____ approach to patient care requires a patient-centered and outcome-oriented way of thinking and acting.
   a. Holistic
   b. Patient care
   c. Goal oriented
   d. Therapeutic

59. Which of the following are included in the psychological domain of Maslow's hierarchy of needs?
   a. Achievement of personal goals
   b. The presence of infection
   c. Respiratory rate
   d. Stress level

60. Which of the following statements would indicate that a surgical technologist is supporting the patient by acknowledging the patient's feelings?
   a. "Everyone is afraid to come to surgery. Just try to relax, and we'll give you some medicine to help you forget you were ever here."
   b. "You say you are afraid. I'll go get you a warm blanket, and then we can talk about it if you'd like."
   c. "I'll go get the surgeon, and you can talk to her about your feelings."
   d. "I'd be afraid, too, if I had your problem and your surgeon."

61. The patient feels greater _____ when team members explain honestly and professionally what is occurring and why.
   a. Security
   b. Fear
   c. Safety
   d. Love

62. Which of the following is NOT common fears found in adult surgical patients?
   a. Fear of pain
   b. Fear of the unknown
   c. Fear of death
   d. Fear of disfigurement

63. Which of the following best describes self-image?
   a. The way we see ourselves in a mirror
   b. The way we think we will look after surgery
   c. The actual way others see us
   d. The way we perceive ourselves in the eyes of others

64. Which of the following describes therapeutic communication?
   a. It is not goal oriented.
   b. It is the same for each patient.
   c. It requires inactive engagement.
   d. It requires good observational skills.

65. The most effective way to approach a patient whose cultural beliefs are different from one's own is with
_____.
   a. An interpreter
   b. A religious person
   c. A different caregiver whose background and beliefs are more similar to those of the patient
   d. Knowledge of that culture

66. _____ is the ability to communicate and interact with people of different cultures and beliefs.
   a. Cultural competence
   b. Cultural awareness
   c. Cultural communication
   d. Belief systems

67. Which of the following ages defines a preschooler?
   a. Birth to 18 months
   b. 19 months to 3 years
   c. 4 to 6 years
   d. 7 to 12 years

68. When communicating with a patient who is impaired:
   a. Speak loudly and use gestures.
   b. Talk only to the caregiver.
   c. Write everything down.
   d. Speak clearly and slowly, facing the patient while talking.

69. Trauma to the body requires _____ during the healing process.
   a. High metabolic activity
   b. Low metabolic activity
   c. Low caloric intake
   d. No change in diet; there are no additional demands

70. In which of the following special populations is your surgical patient most at risk if the person experiences a high volume of blood loss?
   a. Geriatric patients
   b. Mentally challenged
   c. Adolescents
   d. Hearing impaired

71. Which of the following age groups is most sensitive about body image and changes in their body and appearance?
   a. Toddlers
   b. School-age children
   c. Adolescents
   d. Geriatric patients

72. As an age group, _____ welcome explanations and descriptions of how things work and how devices and equipment in the environment relate to their own bodies.
   a. Toddlers
   b. Preschoolers
   c. School-age children
   d. Adolescents

73. Which age group would be likely to view a trip to the hospital and the operating room as punishment?
   a. Infants
   b. Toddlers
   c. Preschoolers
   d. Adolescents

74. Your young patient is being transported to the OR. You find him to be particularly squirmy, and you put extra restraints on him to keep him under control. In which age group would this only increase his terror and resistance?
   a. Infants
   b. Toddlers
   c. Preschoolers
   d. Adolescents

CASE STUDIES

Case Study 1

Read the following case study and answer the questions based on your knowledge of therapeutic communication and geriatric patients.

You have been asked by the OR supervisor to help transport an elderly patient to the preop holding area from her patient room. The patient was recently diagnosed with breast cancer. You enter the patient's room and introduce yourself. The following conversation ensues:

You: "Hello, sweetie. My name is Jane Smith, and I'm here to transport you to surgery today. Can you please tell me the name of your surgeon and the type of procedure you will be having today?"

Mrs. Smith: "Dr. Woods is my surgeon, and he is going to remove my cancer today."

You: "Could you be more specific, Mrs. Smith? Where is your cancer?"

Mrs. Smith:	"The cancer is in my left breast (pause). I'm worried about the surgery. My friend said that the procedure is very disfiguring."
You:	"Many patients are afraid of surgery, Mrs. Smith."
Mrs. Smith:	"I'm worried that I might die from the cancer if the doctor doesn't get it all out."
You:	"Would you like to talk to someone about this before we go to surgery?"
Mrs. Smith:	"No, I guess not. I'm ready to go."
You:	"Okay, can I get you to scoot over to the OR stretcher for me?"

Now answer the following questions about this conversation.

75. Are you comfortable with the way this conversation has gone?

_____

76. Was the conversation helpful in alleviating the patient's fear before you brought her to surgery?

_____

77. Is the conversation you are having with the patient helpful or therapeutic?

_____

78. Go through the conversation and make it therapeutic for the patient. Change your responses above.

Case Study 2

Read the following case study and answer the questions based on your knowledge of patient rights and cultural competency.

In Chapter 2, your textbook states:

Spirituality is a sense or understanding of something more profound than humanity, not perceived by the physical senses.

Patients have the right to express their religious faith in the health care setting.

Examining one's own beliefs and broadening the definition of *spirituality* is the first step toward the development of spiritual care.

Knowing that these statements are true, and evaluating the statement, "Caregivers do not have to have cancer to understand the process," consider this scenario:

You are a CST and your job today in the OR is to assist the circulator with her duties. Your patient arrives in the operating room. He has prayer beads and a religious item that you do not recognize from your own religious practice. You do not know anything about his religion. You are assisting the procedure for a general anesthetic and placing the patient monitors on your patient. He states that he is "afraid" and asks you to pray with him before he goes to sleep.

Answer the following questions about this patient's care.

79. What can you do now to ease his fear?

   _____

   _____

80. Can he keep his religious items with him during the procedure?

   _____

   _____

81. How can you pray with him and still retain your own religious and spiritual beliefs and his as well?

   _____

   _____

82. Evaluate the statement, "Caregivers do not have to have cancer to understand the process" with regard to this patient.

   _____

   _____

Chapter **2** **The Patient in Surgery**

3 Death and Dying

Student's Name _____

KEY TERMS

Write the definition for each term.

1. Coroner's case _____

2. Cultural competence _____

3. Determination of death _____

4. DNAR _____

5. DNR _____

6. Elisabeth Kübler-Ross _____

7. End of life _____

8. Heartbeating cadaver _____

9. Living will _____

10. Livor mortis _____

11. Non-heartbeating cadaver _____

12. Postmortem care _____

13. Required request law _____

14. Rigor mortis _____

15. Self-determination _____

SHORT ANSWERS

Provide a short answer for each question or statement.

16. From a medical point of view, the *end of life* is _____.

17. The reactions of grief and sadness of the surgical patient's family may accompany bouts of _____ with the health system.

18. _____ is the right of every individual to make decisions about how he or she lives and dies.

19. _____ issues arise when decisions about end-of-life care fall to the family when the patient is unable to communicate his or her wishes.

20. _____ or _____ expresses the patient decision to decline life-saving efforts.

21. _____ care is the medical and supportive care provided to the dying patient.

22. Describe briefly the difference between a living will and a DNR order.

_____

_____

MATCHING

Match the term with the correct definition.

23. _____ "If I pray daily, maybe God will allow me
to live."

24. _____ A natural first response, a defense mechanism.

25. _____ The idea that death is no longer a source of
psychological conflict.

26. _____ Refusing nutrition or treatment.

27. _____ "I just want to experience one pain-free
day with my family."

a. Denial

b. Bargaining

c. Anger

d. Acceptance

e. Depression

TRUE/FALSE

Indicate whether the statement is true or false.

28. News of entry into the dying process for oneself or a loved one triggers a cascade of emotional and psychological
events.

_____ True   _____ False

29. When told that they are dying, some patients' first response is to express anger toward the family, themselves, health
workers, or God.

_____ True   _____ False

30. The stages of death are not discrete, nor are they predictable in all people of all cultures.

_____ True   _____ False

31. Many modern models have been developed since Elisabeth Kübler-Ross produced her research in 1960.

_____ True   _____ False

32. When talking with a dying patient, the surgical technologist should avoid communication that attempts to minimize,
rationalize, or deny death.

_____ True   _____ False

33. The most important part of communication when talking to a dying patient is listening to the person.

_____ True   _____ False

34. The surgical technologist may facilitate communication between the family and other professionals but may not discuss medical information directly with the family regarding the patient's condition.

_____ True   _____ False

35. Active measures to prolong life are ethically the same as those that do not halt the progression of death.

_____ True   _____ False

36. Once signed and notarized, the DNR stands as it reads throughout the remainder of the patient's life, with no need for revision.

_____ True   _____ False

37. Patients may refuse treatment at any point in the dying process.

_____ True   _____ False

38. The medical community believes that withdrawal of care constitutes suffering.

_____ True   _____ False

39. If the patient has been ill for some time and no decision has been made, the attending physician must *by law* ask the patient and family to consider organ donation.

_____ True   _____ False

40. Even if health care workers may not agree with the decisions made by their patients or a family member, they are obliged to honor them.

_____ True   _____ False

MULTIPLE CHOICE

Choose the most correct answer to complete the question or statement.

41. Which of the following is a famous physiatrist who constructed the death and dying model that is most frequently recognized today?
    a. Maslow
    b. Freud
    c. Piaget
    d. Elisabeth Kübler-Ross

42. During the dying process, _____ is a defense mechanism that forestalls the full impact of the fact of death until the mind is ready to accept it.
    a. Denial
    b. Acceptance
    c. Bargaining
    d. Anger

43. A dying patient may express anger to _____.
    a. Gain control over the environment
    b. Get even with the physician
    c. Pass through the stages of dying even if the person is not angry
    d. Keep from becoming depressed

44. It is the responsibility of the _____ to convey information about the patient's medical condition to the family and/or friends.
    a. Operating room scheduler or secretary
    b. Surgeon only
    c. Medical and nursing staff
    d. Operating room staff

45. The order to _____ is made official by signing a DNR order, which is charted in the patient's medical record.
   a. Not resuscitate
   b. Call the doctor
   c. Add additional medications
   d. Sign a surgical consent form

46. Examples of palliative care include all of the following *except*:
   a. Debulking of a tumor
   b. X-ray films
   c. Debridement of a pressure wound
   d. Insertion of a gastric feeding tube

47. When a surgical technologist is providing information to family or friends about a patient's medical condition, it is appropriate for the technologist only to:
   a. Report that the surgery is taking longer than usual
   b. Report that the patient is in good hands and is doing well
   c. Offer an acknowledgment of loss
   d. Discuss the laboratory test values

48. The surgical technologist should refrain from providing information to family or friends about _____ of the patient.
   a. A financial report
   b. Counseling
   c. The mental status
   d. The medical condition

49. For surgical technologists to recognize and acknowledge the fact of death and what this means to the patient in that moment and time, they should:
   a. Focus on what the patient is experiencing in the operating room or holding area.
   b. Observe facial expressions and gestures
   c. Be alert to any changes in mood or signs of anxiety and fear related to death and isolation
   d. All of the above

50. Medical interventions for a dying patient include all of the following *except:*
   a. Respiratory support (artificial respiration)
   b. Intravenous feeding
   c. Dialysis
   d. Pain medications

51. The _____ of death is considered by some too constricting and does not allow for individualism in the experience of death.
   a. Stage theory
   b. End of life theory
   c. Spiritual theory
   d. Psychological theory

52. Communication with a dying patient requires keen _____ and observation skills.
   a. Conversational
   b. Written
   c. Listening
   d. Examination

53. The best way to talk to a dying patient is to:
   a. Minimize, rationalize, or deny that the person is dying
   b. Avoid the conversation entirely
   c. Change the subject if the patient brings it up
   d. Talk openly with the patient

54. _____ sometimes is the most effective source of comfort.
   a. Interrupting
   b. Singing
   c. Talking
   d. Listening

55. Family members of a patient who dies suddenly have _____ needs compared with family members of a patient who dies after a lengthy chronic illness.
   a. Different
   b. Similar
   c. Equivalent
   d. Comparable

56. _____ influence the decisions people make about how they want to die or how they would like others to go through the dying process.
   a. Religion
   b. Beliefs
   c. Culture
   d. Both B and C

57. _____ is the right of every individual to make decisions about how he or she lives and dies.
   a. DNR
   b. Advance directive
   c. Self-determination
   d. Living will

58. A _____ specifies the exact nature of palliative care that a patient accepts.
   a. Living will
   b. Advance directive
   c. DNR
   d. Assisted suicide

59. When no verifiable permission has been granted for organ donation by the patient, the _____ may act as a surrogate for the patient.
   a. Surgeon
   b. Family
   c. Chaplain
   d. Nurses

60. In the operating room, death is a(n) _____
    event.
    a. Rare
    b. Occasional
    c. Weekly
    d. Daily

CASE STUDIES

Case Study 1

Read the following case study and answer the questions based on your knowledge of death and dying.

You are scrubbed in on a local breast biopsy, and your patient is under conscious sedation. The surgeon removes the breast lump and says to you out loud, "This is not good. This patient has cancer." After a very brief silence, he says, "I'll have to schedule her for a mastectomy for next week." You close the wound, and as the patient emerges from the sedation, she asks you how the procedure turned out.

61. What can you tell the patient about her condition?

    _____

    _____

62. If you do not disclose to the patient what the surgeon said, are you lying to the patient?

    _____

    _____

63. If you do disclose to the patient what the surgeon said, are you breaking a confidence?

    _____

    _____

INTERNET EXERCISES

Internet Exercise 1

*Using your favorite search engine and the key words **organ donation**, go online and look for the nearest organ donation system. Answer the following questions about organ donation.*

64. Where is the donation system nearest to where you live?

    _____

    _____

65. How many miles away is that?

_____

_____

66. Did you find guidelines for organ donation listed on the Web site?

_____

_____

Internet Exercise 2

Do an Internet search using the key words **organ donor**. _Look for guidelines for becoming an organ donor. (You do not have to become a donor, you just have to research the idea.)_

67. Are there organ donation forms that you could download and sign to become an organ donor?

_____

_____

68. What are the guidelines?

_____

_____

69. What should you discuss with your family members to make sure that your wishes about organ donation are executed as you instructed?

_____

_____

4 Law and Ethics

Student's Name _____

KEY TERMS

Write the definition for each term.

1. Abandonment _____

2. Administrative law _____

3. Advance directive _____

4. Court trial _____

5. Damages _____

6. Defamation _____

7. Delegation _____

8. Deposition _____

9. Ethics _____

10. Ethical dilemma _____

11. Informed consent _____

12. Insurance _____

13. Jury trial _____

14. Impairment (cognitive) _____

15. Laws _____

16. Liable _____

17. Libel _____

18. Living will _____

19. Malpractice _____

20. Medical ethics _____

21. Medical power of attorney _____

22. Negligence _____

23. Operative report _____

24. Perjury _____

25. Professional ethics _____

26. Professional license _____

27. Punitive _____

28. Retained object _____

29. Sentinel event _____

30. Sexual harassment _____

31. Slander _____

32. Statutes _____

33. Subpoena _____

34. Summons _____

35. Time out _____

36. Tort _____

SHORT ANSWERS

Provide a short answer for each question or statement.

37. Legal boundaries for the surgical technologist are defined by *what is not permitted* rather than by *what is permitted*. What is NOT permitted?

_____

_____

38. Honoring the patient's privacy is a standard of conduct established by all health professions. This is a part of the code of conduct for hospitals. What are other standards of practice for surgical technologists?

_____

_____

39. What are the legal and ethical problems when a person delegating a task requests a task that the delegatee cannot or should not perform?

_____

_____

40. What is accountability in the practice of surgical technology if the certified surgical technologist is always to work under the direct supervision of a registered or licensed person?

_____

_____

41. What does the Latin phrase *respondeat superior* mean?

_____

_____

42. Certain cases of negligence are so evident that there can be no defense, or no further information is needed to prove the negligence. What is the Latin term for this concept? How does the term work into a case of negligence?

_____

_____

43. In legal terms, what does it mean for a person to "do no harm"? Contrast that with what it means to the operating room team to "do no harm." Are they the same?

_____

_____

44. How is it that the legal term for "borrowed servants" no longer applies to modern hospitals and surgery centers?

_____

_____

_____

45. What is the difference between an intentional tort and an unintentional tort?

_____

_____

46. What are the four elements of negligence that must be proven in a lawsuit?

_____

_____

47. Give two examples of a negligent burn that may occur in the operating room suite.

_____

_____

48. When working in the operating room, what is the best way to reduce or avoid the risk of harm to others?

_____

_____

_____

Chapter **4** **Law and Ethics**

49. When is it appropriate for a practicing surgical technologist to question and/or refuse an assignment in the operating room without ethical and moral questions arising about the technologist's practice?

_____

_____

_____

_____

MATCHING I

Match each term with the correct definition.

50. _____ Regulates the use of chemicals for disinfection and sterilization

51. _____ Issues and enforces standards for the protection of employees and patients

52. _____ Laws that protect the public from medical devices

53. _____ Laws that differ from state to state

54. _____ Manual that describes safe practices and policies, such as infection control, aseptic technique, and disinfection and sterilization methods

55. _____ Manual that describes the general administrative and logistical operations of the hospital

56. _____ Allows nurses to administer medications prescribed by a physician

57. _____ A law that requires hospitals to report any incident in which a medical device is believed to be the cause of an injury or death

58. _____ Rules that pertain to how people behave, which are based on the principles that the organization values

a. OSHA

b. EPA

c. FDA

d. Safe Medical Device Act

e. Nurse Practice Act

f. Hospital policy

g. Operating room procedure manual

h. State laws

i. Standard of conduct

TRUE/FALSE

Indicate whether the statement is true or false.

59. Surgical technologists are guided in their practice by society's rules and laws.

_____ True   _____ False

60. Because a certified surgical technologist is unlicensed, his or her actions are judged according to civil or criminal law, as are those of any other person in society.

_____ True   _____ False

61. Legal boundaries for the surgical technologist are defined by *what is not permitted*.

_____ True   _____ False

62. Accredited hospitals and other health care facilities are not required to orient new employees.

_____ True   _____ False

63. Forgetting to read about policy or protocol changes does not protect an employee from legal action in case of negligence.

_____ True   _____ False

64. Delegation of duties in health care settings is an infrequent occurrence.

_____ True   _____ False

65. Accountability for a retained object lies only with the surgical technologist.

_____ True   _____ False

66. Negligent torts are the most common example of tort liability in the health care setting.

_____ True   _____ False

67. Surgical personnel are ethically and legally obligated to remain on the job until relieved by another staff member, even if they have been there for many hours.

_____ True   _____ False

68. Patients may refuse blood or tissue products because of their faith or personal beliefs.

_____ True   _____ False

MATCHING II

Match the term to the correct description. Some terms are used more than once.

69. _____ The supreme law of the nation or the state

70. _____ Bills passed by state legislatures and signed into law by the governor

71. _____ Laws passed by legislative bodies

72. _____ Laws created by agencies and bodies of the government

73. _____ Rules established by the EPA for the handling of medical waste

74. _____ Rulings issued by courts that have the effect of law and are binding (legal)

75. _____ A state board of practice that establishes standards for practice

76. _____ Established laws that govern the actions of those in a given profession

77. _____ Based on precedence from previous cases

78. _____ Laws acted upon by OSHA

a. Constitutional law
b. Statues
c. Administrative law
d. Common law
e. Professional practice acts

Choose the correct answer for the question or statement.

79. Which of the following would NOT be considered an unintentional tort?
    a. Retained object
    b. Improper positioning
    c. Incorrect operative site
    d. Invasion of privacy

80. Which of the following statements about positioning of the surgical patient is true?
    a. Only those who are specifically trained and competent to position the patient should assist in this task.
    b. Anyone in the operating room can help position a surgical patient.
    c. Only the surgeon should position the surgical patient.
    d. Once the patient is under general anesthesia, the anesthesiologist is responsible for the individual's final position.

81. Which of the following is NOT a potential injury caused by improper patient positioning?
    a. Underextension of limbs
    b. Pressure on bony prominences
    c. Loss of circulation
    d. Improper ventilation

82. The main reasons for making an incident report after an accident or incident is/are:
    a. For quality assurance
    b. To increase the risk of the hospital
    c. To protect the hospital from lawyers
    d. All of the above

CASE STUDIES

Case Study 1

Read the following case study and answer the questions based on your knowledge of unintentional torts or civil wrongs.

You have just been served with legal documents that suggest that you were scrubbed in on a procedure in which your patient was burned. You are charged with negligence. What are the possible causes of the burn?

1. _____
2. _____
3. _____
4. _____
5. _____
6. _____
7. _____
8. _____
9. _____

Case Study 2

Read through the following case study. The areas of the scenario that are numbered and italicized are areas of potential negligence if the duties are not performed correctly. Write a brief sentence about each of the numbered and italicized areas to describe which area of civil or criminal liability applies.

Your patient is being transported to the preanesthesia unit (PAU) by the transport team. The patient is accompanied by her neighbor, who will drive the patient home after the procedure.

When the team gets to the PAU, the room is empty. The transport team *(1) leaves the patient and (2) the chart* in the room to search for the nurse in charge. When the nurse gets to the room, she sedates the patient, as ordered on the chart by the anesthesiologist. The nurse notices that the patient has several necklaces on. She knows that the patient should not go into surgery wearing these, so she asks the patient to *(3) remove the necklaces*. She puts them loosely on the end of the patient's bed.

The nurse has been in the room for about 20 minutes and needs to check on the lab results. She asks a high school nurse's aide student *(4) to stand in the room* with the patient while she is gone. The aide is instructed to "holler for help" if she needs something.

When the nurse returns to the room, she notices that the consent form has not been signed. She *(5) asks the patient to sign the consent,* and *(6) asks the nurse's aide to witness.*

(1) _____

(2) _____

(3) _____

(4) _____

(5) _____

(6) _____

INTERNET EXERCISES

Internet Exercise 1

Go online and search for operating room legal issues that would apply to the term **res ipsa loquitur**. *These lawsuits not only are easy to find, they are particularly ridiculous, because if a competent, organized, and conscientious surgical team had been present, they would never have filed. Briefly describe one of the lawsuits and then explain how the incident could have been avoided. Remember to cite your Internet reference.*

_____

_____

_____

_____

_____

Reference: _____

Internet Exercise 2

Using your favorite search engine and the keywords **medical ethics,** *find a journal article on the subject. Make a report appropriate to present to your class and include the following information.*

1. Internet site reference

2. Date of access

3. Title of the journal

4. Author and title of the article

5. What medical ethic was discussed?

6. Was a lawsuit involved?

7. What conclusion was given at the end of the article?

5 Introduction to the Health Care Facility

Student's Name _____

KEY TERMS

Write the definition for each term.

1. Accreditation _____

2. Air exchange _____

3. Biomedical technologist _____

4. Case cart system _____

5. Central core _____

6. Chain of command _____

7. Contaminated _____

8. Decontamination area _____

9. Efficiency _____

10. High-efficiency particulate air (HEPA) filters _____

11. Laminar airflow (LAF) system _____

12. Mission statement _____

13. Organizational chart (Organigram) _____

14. OSHA _____

15. Personnel policy _____

16. Postanesthesia care unit (PACU) _____

17. Restricted area _____

18. Risk management _____

19. Role confusion _____

20. Satellite facilities _____

21. Semirestricted area _____

22. Traffic patterns _____

23. Transitional area _____

24. Unrestricted area _____

Provide a short answer for each question or statement.

25. The surgical department is structured and engineered with three objectives in mind. What are they?

    a. _____

    b. _____

    c. _____

26. Traffic patterns in the operating room are restricted. Describe the typical traffic pattern for an operating room and explain why the movement is restricted.

    _____

    _____

    _____

    _____

27. Explain how the airflow in the operating room is directed to prevent infection.

    _____

    _____

    _____

28. What is the difference between a LAF system and a HEPA system?

    _____

    _____

    _____

29. Instruments that are particularly delicate and expensive (e.g., an eye tray) might not go to the sterile processing room. What is a more appropriate way to process instruments such as these after a surgical procedure?

    _____

    _____

30. What physiological risks does your patient face when admitted to the PACU?

    _____

    _____

    _____

31. The operating room could not function without the collaborative efforts of professionals outside the OR. Which other departments collaborate with the OR?

a. _____

b. _____

c. _____

d. _____

e. _____

f. _____

g. _____

h. _____

i. _____

j. _____

k. _____

l. _____

m. _____

n. _____

32. Surgery is performed in many different settings. What are they?

_____

_____

_____

_____

_____

33. Surgery that requires _____ is performed in a hospital facility.

34. Who is the operating room educator, and what are the job duties of this person in the operating room?

_____

_____

_____

35. Explain how the chain of command and the organizational chart are interrelated.

_____

_____

_____

_____

MATCHING

Match each term with the correct definition. Some terms may be used more than once.

36. _____ Includes a firm pad to help make the patient comfortable

37. _____ A large, stainless steel table on which all instruments and supplies are placed

38. _____ After gowning and gloving, the scrub arranges all the equipment in an orderly manner

39. _____ The table is placed over or alongside the patient for quick access to instruments

40. _____ May hold the surgical patient prep or electrical equipment

41. _____ Sterile water or saline are distributed into this

42. _____ Designated for soiled surgical sponges

43. _____ Covered with a sterile drape and used to hold instruments and supplies that are immediately required during surgery

a. Mayo stand
b. Back table
c. Operating table
d. Kick bucket
e. Ring stand/basin
f. Prep table

TRUE/FALSE

Indicate whether the statement is true or false.

44. Infection control involves many different areas of expertise and practice.

_____ True   _____ False

45. In an emergency, time sometimes is the most important factor in achieving a good outcome.

_____ True   _____ False

46. The primary design goal of the operating suite floor plan is to create a clear separation between soiled and clean equipment.

_____ True   _____ False

47. Allowing airflow from restricted to unrestricted areas poses no infection risk to patients.

_____ True   _____ False

48. Static electricity is a fire hazard in the operating room only because of the presence of anesthetic inhalation agents.

_____ True   _____ False

49. The operating room suite must be maintained at 50% to 55% total humidity.

_____ True   _____ False

50. The integrated OR allows the surgeon to control surgical devices and equipment through a foot-activated system.

_____ True   _____ False

51. Regardless of the type of procedure or how urgent the case is, the patient is always admitted to the preoperative holding area before surgery.

_____ True   _____ False

52. Accreditation implies a high standard of care and commitment to public safety and welfare.

_____ True   _____ False

53. An organizational chart is a graphic representation of the management chain of command.

_____ True   _____ False

54. The central processing or sterile processing technician is responsible for the safe management only of equipment used in surgery.

_____ True   _____ False

55. Laws concerning the practice of medicine, nursing, and allied health have been established to protect the public.

_____ True   _____ False

56. The chain of command is a relationship between management and the staff.

_____ True   _____ False

MULTIPLE CHOICE

Choose the most correct answer to complete the question or statement.

57. The air in the surgical suite is contained by keeping the doors closed and maintaining higher air pressure inside the suite than outside because _____.
   a. The air outside the suite cannot be completely separated from the air inside the suite.
   b. The air outside the suite is unsterile.
   c. The air inside the suite is dust free.
   d. The air in the hospital is full of airborne bacteria and is considered contaminated.

58. To reduce the risk of infection, air pressure in the surgical suite is maintained at a level _____ higher than the air pressure in adjacent semirestricted areas.
   a. 5%
   b. 8%
   c. 10%
   d. 12%

59. _____ forces air from the operating room into the hallways.
   a. Negative pressure
   b. Equal pressure
   c. Positive pressure
   d. Equivalent pressure

60. The operating room suite must be maintained at _____ relative humidity.
   a. 40% to 45%
   b. 50% to 55%
   c. 50% to 60%
   d. 60% to 65%

61. The surgical lights usually are halogen lamps, which emit a light that is _____.
   a. Very pale blue
   b. Light pink
   c. Bright white
   d. Nonglare white

62. Which of the following operating rooms would be designated a "special procedure" room?
   a. ENT
   b. Neuro
   c. Exploratory laparotomy
   d. Cystoscopy

63. A integrated OR allows the surgeon to activate which of the following surgical devices?
   a. Endoscopic controls
   b. Volume of music
   c. Surgeon's beeper
   d. Computer and communication devices

64. The _____ is a check-in point where the surgeon, anesthesiologist, and circulating nurse can confirm that all laboratory and preoperative documentation is in order.
   a. Scrub sink area
   b. Preoperative holding area
   c. Postoperative recovery area
   d. Surgical offices

65. This area may hold sterile supplies or a flash sterilizer.
   a. Scrub sink area
   b. Preoperative holding area
   c. Substerile room
   d. Instrument holding area

66. Wrapped and sterile operating room supplies may be stored in designated restricted areas adjacent to the operating suites nearby; these areas are called the _____.
   a. Sterile instrument room
   b. Equipment storage area
   c. Substerile room
   d. Utility/workroom

67. Soiled instruments and equipment are _____ and washed in a utility workroom or central processing area.
   a. Sterilized
   b. Rinsed
   c. Decontaminated
   d. Sorted

68. This area must be contained and must be away from all restricted areas to prevent cross-contamination of sterile and clean equipment and supplies.
   a. Sterile instrument room
   b. Utility/workroom
   c. Substerile room
   d. Operating room

69. After surgery, soiled instruments and equipment are decontaminated and then assembled in trays, wrapped, and _____.
   a. Sent to central sterile processing
   b. Resterilized
   c. Disinfected
   d. Sorted

70. The anesthesia workroom is considered a _____ area.
   a. Restricted
   b. Semirestricted
   c. Decontamination
   d. Nonrestricted

71. Physical barriers and procedures necessary in the operating room to maintain strict asepsis also _____ the environment for the staff.
   a. Isolate
   b. Sterilize
   c. Disinfect
   d. Constrict

72. The Joint Commission (TJC) requires that all hospital policies be available to staff members in written form; these are called _____.
   a. MSDS sheets
   b. Principles
   c. Hospital policy
   d. TJC rules

73. Health care facilities and institutions in the United States are accredited by:
   a. TJC
   b. AORN
   c. OSHA
   d. ARC-ST

Case Study 1

Read the following case study and, using the information given, fill in the organizational chart provided.

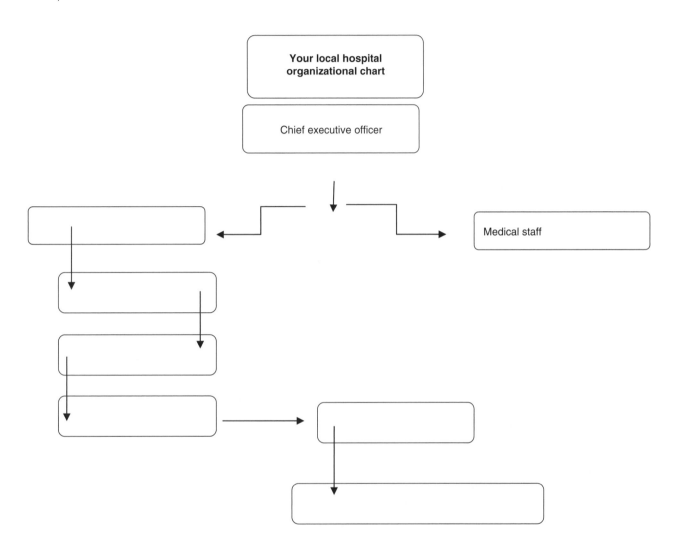

You have just been hired at your local hospital. Mr. Hall is the chief administrator. He has also just been hired. He asks you if you could show him the chain of command for your area of surgical services. Because you work in a very small hospital, there are only two certified surgical technologists, you and one other scrub (Jane). Two nurses (Judy and Jennifer) work in the OR. When you are scrubbed, you work mostly with Dr. May and Dr. Smith.

The charge nurse for your area is Mrs. Jones. She has worked at the hospital in this position for 25 years. The operating room staff educator's name is Jo. Mrs. Markus is the operating room nurse manager, and she reports to the director of perioperative services. His name is Mr. Smith. Mr. Smith reports to the vice president of patient care services, Mr. Zander.

Internet Exercise 1

Go online and research the design of operating rooms. In the space provided, draw a typical design. Include areas of restriction and use colored pencils to color code them. Be creative, but make sure to include all areas of the operating room suite to make it functional.

Internet Exercise 2

Now that you have drawn the entire suite, draw the operating room itself. Using the phrase from your text, **"everything in its place, and a place for everything,"** *put all of the following items in your OR:*

- Anesthesia machine and patient monitors
- Trash/linen hampers
- Back table
- Mayo stand
- Ring stands
- Operating table with arm boards
- Kick bucket
- Computer/communication station
- Prep table
- Closed storage units
- ESU

After you have drawn in all the critical items in your operating room, compare it to your learning space at your school of instruction. How does it compare? Are there critical items that you would like to see in the lab? If so, list them:

_____

_____

6   Communication and Teamwork

Student's Name _____

KEY TERMS

Write the definition for each term.

1. Aggression _____
2. Assertiveness _____
3. Body language _____
4. Consensus _____
5. Content _____
6. Gossip _____
7. Groupthink _____
8. Message _____
9. Norms _____
10. Therapeutic touch _____
11. Tone _____
12. Values _____
13. Win-lose solution _____

SHORT ANSWERS

Provide a short answer for each question or statement.

14. The operating room environment is stressful and includes long hours, insufficient breaks, low pay, and sometimes verbal abuse, which can result in loss of morale and may lead to burnout. This downward spiral can be prevented. What have you learned about how to avoid burnout?

_____

_____

_____

_____

15. When we speak as we would like to be spoken to, we are:

_____

_____

16. Briefly explain the phrase "touch is almost never neutral." _____

    _____

    _____

17. _____ is a privilege earned by trust and limited by the boundaries of culture and social custom.

18. _____ is purposeful touch that conveys empathy, tenderness, and care.

19. Allowing others to think carefully before speaking shows _____.

20. What are the elements of positive listening skills?

    a.

    b.

    c.

    d.

    e.

    f.

    g.

    h.

    i.

21. In the operating room, where communication often is rushed, the sender should look for _____ or body language in the receiver to make sure the message has been received.

22. What environmental barriers to good communication are common in the operating room?

    _____

    _____

    _____

23. How is feedback given?

    _____

    _____

    _____

24. Many people begin to formulate a response before they have heard everything the sender has to say. Their thoughts are focused on what they want to say, and they fail to receive the message. What can you do to make sure you have been heard?

_____

_____

_____

_____

MATCHING

Match each term with the correct definition regarding communication. Some terms may be used more than once.

25. _____ The person who expresses ideas and feelings

26. _____ Phone calls

27. _____ The processor of the message and provider of feedback

28. _____ A response by the receiver that acknowledges the message that was sent

29. _____ The concept, thought, or idea expressed

30. _____ The way the message is expressed

31. _____ The environment of the message

32. _____ Face-to-face discussions

33. _____ Facial expression, body movement, and tone of voice

34. _____ Verbal and nonverbal

35. _____ The actual information conveyed in a communication

a. Sender
b. Receiver
c. Message
d. Feedback
e. Delivery
f. Verbal communication
g. Tone

TRUE/FALSE

Indicate whether the statement is true or false.

36. Good communication requires active participation and a willingness to work with others for the common goal.

_____ True   _____ False

37. In the health care setting, the exchange of information is a primary responsibility for every staff member.

_____ True   _____ False

38. Communication requires only a sender or a receiver.

_____ True   _____ False

39. Verbal communication means only communication that is spoken.

_____ True   _____ False

40. The tone of the dialogue reflects the sender's emotions.

_____ True   _____ False

41. Touch can be an expression of comfort and is almost never neutral.

_____ True   _____ False

42. Listening requires active participation.

_____ True   _____ False

43. The assertive person puts his or her own needs and wants above those of everyone else.

_____ True   _____ False

44. People do not immediately sense when another person respects them; the respect has to be earned repeatedly through their actions.

_____ True   _____ False

45. Respectful people disparage other people to appear smarter, more skilled, or "better."

_____ True   _____ False

46. Deliberately withholding information from a person that could affect the individual's work is considered sabotage.

_____ True   _____ False

47. The most powerful way to instill civility in a group is to model it.

_____ True   _____ False

48. Most role confusion is a result of good communication skills.

_____ True   _____ False

49. Economic communication is the same as withholding information.

_____ True   _____ False

Choose the most correct answer to complete the question or statement.

50. _____ is the ability to express one's own needs and rights while respecting the needs and rights of others.
    a. Listening
    b. Criticism
    c. Collaboration
    d. Assertiveness

51. Which of the following is NOT one of the elements of good communication?
    a. Feedback
    b. Sender
    c. Receiver
    d. Delivery

52. _____ are based on tradition and value systems.
    a. Social practice
    b. Values
    c. Norms
    d. Cultural beliefs

53. Qualities of good listening skills include all of the following *except* _____ .
    a. Listening
    b. Social practice
    c. Assertiveness
    d. Respect

54. _____ frequently lead(s) to inaccurate interpretation or to inability to respond to the information.
    a. Positive listening skills
    b. Passive listening
    c. Talking
    d. Active listening

55. Which of the following kinds of body language shows assertiveness?
    a. Good posture
    b. Eye contact, including a fixed stare
    c. Fidgeting and shifting your weight from foot to foot
    d. Interrupting

56. Revealing personal or confidential information about others is _____.
    a. Disrespectful
    b. Trustworthy
    c. Demanding of others' attention
    d. Judgmental

57. Poor communication results when a message is delivered but the receiver does not acknowledge understanding. In this case, there is no _____.
    a. Message
    b. Feedback
    c. Receiver
    d. Code

58. A person who is respectful _____.
    a. Interrupts
    b. Demands attention
    c. Responds with empathy
    d. Judges and gossips about others

59. Because the work environment is intense, your own intensity has an effect on others; therefore, even if you are emotionally upset, you should _____ before you begin a conversation.
    a. Talk to someone else as a practice
    b. Yell as loudly as possible
    c. Calm down
    d. Ask for advice from a coworker

60. Which of the following is NOT a way that communication might fail?
    a. False perception
    b. Assumptions
    c. Bias
    d. Understanding

61. Which of the following is NOT a common stressor for work in the operating room?
    a. The social structure in the operating room is undergoing a change.
    b. Surgeons might be competing for staff members or for operating room times.
    c. The unit is friendly and unrushed.
    d. Teamwork is needed, even if the members are not friends.

62. Which of the following is considered the primary behavior problem in the OR?
    a. Verbal abuse
    b. Mental abuse
    c. Power misuse
    d. Miscommunication

63. When verbal abuse is reported and the administration does little to address or act on the problem in a serious manner, _____ occurs.
    a. Escalation
    b. Implied permission
    c. Deceleration
    d. Communication

64. _____ is/are one of the most effective ways to counteract verbal abuse.
   a. Vulgar responses
   b. Teamwork
   c. Assertive behavior
   d. Aggressive behavior

65. Which of the following is a true statement about gossiping?
   a. It is insidious behavior that hurts people, erodes teamwork, and damages group ethics.
   b. It is the same as the normal sharing of news or events that occur in people's lives.
   c. It is communication about another person or event that is nonconfidential.
   d. As gossip spreads, the story may change slightly.

66. Groupthink _____.
   a. is based on the idea that each individual will have his or her own ideas and processes
   b. is noncollective behavior and thinking
   c. produces two types of people: those who are in, and those who are out
   d. usually is a positive force because it allows for freedom of speech

67. When criticism is used to exercise power over others or to boost one's self-confidence, it can be _____.
   a. Very destructive
   b. A positive experience
   c. A good learning experience for students
   d. An aid to agreement

68. Any act that evokes humiliation, shame, or guilt should be reported as _____.
   a. Aggressive behavior
   b. Sexual harassment
   c. Teamwork
   d. Assertive behavior

69. The _____ is only one type of team that plans and implements patient care in the operating room.
   a. Surgical team
   b. Surgeon
   c. Nursing staff
   d. Anesthesiologist

70. A business model for teamwork, developed in the 1960s by Bruce Tuckman, was based on four group processes. Which of the following is NOT one of his four groups?
   a. Brainforming
   b. Storming
   c. Norming
   d. Performing

71. Speaking with others in an even and calm manner without sarcasm promotes _____.
   a. Anger as a response
   b. Aggressiveness
   c. Retreat of coworkers
   d. Stress reduction

72. Collaboration:
   a. Requires that everyone solve problems and obstacles as a group
   b. Is the most powerful way to instill civility in a group
   c. Identifies new tasks or procedures and implements them with as little disruption as possible
   d. Causes members to feel frustrated

73. _____ occurs when individuals are uncertain of what is expected of them.
   a. Assertiveness
   b. Teamwork
   c. Collaboration
   d. Role confusion

74. Positive listening skills include all of the following rules *except* _____.
   a. Focus on the receiver.
   b. Avoid listening for what you want to hear.
   c. Watch for nonverbal cues.
   d. Ask for clarification.

Case Study 1

Study Table 6-1, on body language, in your text. Go to a public area (e.g., a classroom, the library, the mall) and take notes on the body language of someone across from you. As you observe the person, try to notice 10 different types of body language. In the following chart, list the element of body language and what it commonly demonstrates.

Element of body language	What it demonstrates
1.	
2.	
3.	
4.	
5.	
6.	
7.	
8.	
9.	
10.	

Where were you located as you watched the person? _____.

Case Study 2

Read the following scenario and then answer the questions that follow.

You are in the operating room and scrubbed in for an exploratory laparotomy. The anesthesiologist and your circulator are chatting about a movie they both recently saw. Your surgeon is not talking, and you notice that the surgeon has started to become anxious and increasingly more difficult to work with. The surgeon says that this is becoming a difficult case and asks you to hold a retractor.

You continue with your job, and when the patient begins to bleed more than normal, you ask your circulator to turn off the music. The surgeon gets the bleeding under control, and you finish the case.

After the patient has been taken to the PACU and is stable, your circulator comes to you and asks to talk to you about being "snotty" during the procedure. She suggests that you made her look "stupid" in front of the surgeon and the anesthesiologist.

75. What social cues might your surgeon have started to show that caused you to think she was getting anxious?

_____

_____

76. By turning off the music, you have reduced some of the environmental barriers that are present in the operating room. What are others that you could change?

_____

_____

77. Your circulator has a perception that you were being "snotty" during the procedure. What can you do to change her perception of what happened?

_____

_____

_____

_____

INTERNET EXERCISES

Internet Exercise 1

Using your favorite Internet search engine and the keyword teamwork, find two sites that describe good teamwork skills.

78. What type of suggestions do the sites offer for fostering good teamwork?

_____

_____

_____

_____

79. Do the sites you chose include information on how to deal with difficult personalities? What are some measures they recommend for the conditions cited?

_____

_____

_____

80. What two sites did you use?

    a. www._____

    b. www._____

Internet Exercise 2

Using your favorite Internet search engine, search for a journal article that deals with conflict resolution and good communication skills. This article does not need to be about a conflict in the operating room, it just needs to be about a conflict. After you have read the article, provide the following information:

81. What was the title of the article? _____

    _____

82. List the author(s) _____

    _____

83. What was the conflict described in the article? _____

    _____

    _____

    _____

84. Was the article fact or fiction? _____

85. How was the conflict resolved?_____

    _____

    _____

86. How would you have handled the conflict differently? _____

    _____

    _____

    _____

    _____

7 Microbes and the Process of Infection

Student's Name _____

KEY TERMS

Write the definition for each term.

1. Acquired immunity _____
2. Aerobe _____
3. Aerosol droplet _____
4. Anaerobe _____
5. Anaphylactic shock _____
6. Antibiotic _____
7. Antibiotic resistant _____
8. Antibodies _____
9. Antigens _____
10. Autoinfection _____
11. Bacilli _____
12. Bacteria (pl.); bacterium (sing.) _____
13. Bacteriology _____
14. Bacteriophage _____
15. Bioburden _____
16. Capsule _____
17. Carrier _____
18. Cocci _____
19. Colonization _____
20. Commensalism _____
21. Community-acquired infection _____
22. Contaminated _____
23. Cross-contamination _____
24. Culture _____
25. Culture and sensitivity _____
26. Dehiscence _____
27. Direct transmission _____

28. Droplet nuclei _____

29. Endospore (spore) _____

30. Endotoxin _____

31. Entry site _____

32. Evisceration _____

33. Exotoxin _____

34. Facultative _____

35. Fomite _____

36. Gram stain _____

37. Host _____

38. Infection _____

39. Inflammation _____

40. Immunity _____

41. Lysogenesis _____

42. Mycotic _____

43. Nonpathogenic _____

44. Nosocomial infection _____

45. Nucleolus _____

46. Opportunistic _____

47. Osmosis _____

48. Pathogen _____

49. Pathogenicity _____

50. Pathology _____

51. Phagocyte _____

52. Phagocytosis _____

53. Pili _____

54. Prion _____

55. Resident microorganisms _____

56. Spirochete _____

57. Spore _____

58. Staining _____

59. Standard Precautions _____

60. Sterile _____

61. Vacuole _____

LABELING

Label the following drawing of a prokaryotic cell. Make sure to use medical terminology where appropriate.

62.

63.

64.

65.

66.

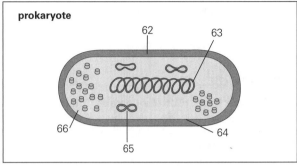

Modified from Goering R, Dockrell H, Wakelin D et al: *Mim's microbiology*, ed 4, St Louis, 2008, Mosby

Label the following drawing of a eukaryotic cell. Make sure to use medical terminology where appropriate.

67.

68.

69.

70.

71.

72.

73.

74.

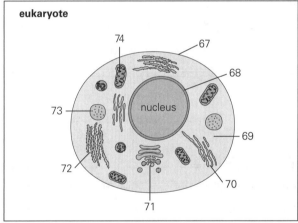

Modified from Goering R, Dockrell H, Wakelin D et al: *Mim's microbiology*, ed 4, St Louis, 2008, Mosby

SHORT ANSWERS

Provide a short answer for each question or statement.

75. One of the first classification systems was developed approximately 300 years ago and is called

the ＿＿＿＿＿＿＿＿＿＿＿ system.

76. An example of a natural body defense of the human eye is ＿＿＿＿＿＿＿＿＿.

77. ＿＿＿＿＿＿＿＿＿ develops when the body is stimulated to form its own antibodies against specific disease antigens.

78. Inoculating a culture plate with a microbe and placing small paper disks impregnated with various antibacterial

agents on the sample is called a(an) ＿＿＿＿＿＿＿＿＿.

79. Gram staining is routinely performed to differentiate bacteria into two primary classifications:

_____ and _____.

80. Rod-shaped bacilli occur singly or in _____.

81. _____ are chemicals contained within the cell wall of bacteria.

MATCHING I

Match each term with the correct definition.

82. _____ Cellular organism lacking a true nucleus

83. _____ Group that includes only bacteria and the Archaea

84. _____ Organism with a characteristic cell surrounded by a membrane

85. _____ Organism containing complex organs for metabolism and reproduction

86. _____ Living organism

87. _____ Organism with a cell wall

88. _____ Cellular organism lacking a nuclear membrane

a. Prokaryote
b. Eukaryote
c. Both

MATCHING II

Match each term with the correct definition regarding microbial relationships.

89. _____ One organism is harmed, and the other benefits.

90. _____ Two organisms of different species live together.

91. _____ Two organisms exist in a state that benefits both.

92. _____ Two organisms exist in a state in which neither is harmed.

a. Symbiosis
b. Commensalism
c. Mutualism
d. Parasitism

TRUE/FALSE

Indicate whether the sentence or statement is true or false.

93. Medical microbiology is the study of microscopic animal and plant organisms.

_____ True   _____ False

94. A commonly used taxonomy system in biology has seven categories or classifications.

_____ True   _____ False

95. The cell theory developed in the early 1600s formed the basis of biological study and is still referred to today.

_____ True   _____ False

96. The only true organelle of the prokaryote is the ribosome, which synthesizes protein.

_____ True   _____ False

97. All microorganisms are considered pathogenic.

_____ True   _____ False

60

98. The Gram staining procedure requires two dyes.

_____ True   _____ False

99. Identification of the shape and size of bacteria is insufficient to identify the exact species.

_____ True   _____ False

100. The microscope is a delicate and expensive instrument with numerous components.

_____ True   _____ False

101. Anaerobic bacteria can live with or without oxygen.

_____ True   _____ False

102. The endospore is a dormant phase in the reproductive cycle in which bacteria form a thick, multilayered protein wall around their genetic material.

_____ True   _____ False

MULTIPLE CHOICE

Choose the most correct answer to complete the question or statement.

103. Virology is the study of:
    a. Disease mechanisms, diagnosis, and treatment
    b. Bacteria
    c. Microbes
    d. Viruses

104. The Linnean system divides living things into either _____, according to evolutionary descent.
    a. Plant or animal
    b. Mineral or animal
    c. Vegetable or animal
    d. Genus and species

105. Which of the following categories is NOT included in the Linnean system of taxonomy?
    a. Domain
    b. Order
    c. Brothers
    d. Phylum

106. Which of the following is NOT a characteristic of eukaryotic cells?
    a. Multicellular
    b. Double-layer membrane
    c. Cell membrane
    d. Include bacteria and Archaea

107. The primary structural difference between the prokaryote and eukaryote is:
    a. Prokaryotes are more like human cells.
    b. Prokaryotes have a semipermeable cell membrane.
    c. Prokaryotes have no distinct nucleus.
    d. Eukaryotes are not pathogenic.

108. The _____ protects the cell from drying and provides resistance to chemicals and invasion by viruses.
    a. Cell wall
    b. Capsule
    c. Cell membrane
    d. Spores

109. The _____ is also called the slime layer.
    a. Cell wall
    b. Cell membrane
    c. Outside layer of the nucleus
    d. Capsule

110. _____ is a process in which the cell engulfs large particles from outside the cell.
    a. Phagocytosis
    b. Pinocytosis
    c. Active transport
    d. Endocytosis

111. The human intestinal tract contains many different types of bacteria, such as *Escherichia coli,* which are essential for metabolism. This is an example of _____ .
    a. Mutualism
    b. Parasitism
    c. Symbiosis
    d. Commensalism

112. Which of the following exams are used to test for tuberculosis?
    a. Gram staining
    b. Culture
    c. Sensitivity
    d. Acid-fast

CASE STUDIES

Case Study 1

Read the following case study and answer the questions based on your knowledge of classification of surgical wounds.

You are scheduled for trauma call, and you get called in for a patient who was performing in a rodeo. He fell off his horse and is being admitted for an open fracture of the femur. Use Table 7-3 in your text to answer the following questions.

113. How would this be classified?

114. What is this patient's risk for infection?

115. If the wound were not open and the patient were admitted for a femoral fracture, how would the wound be classified?

Case Study 2

Read the following case study and answer the questions based on your knowledge of identification of microorganisms.

You are in the operating room and scrubbed in. Your surgeon opens the patient's stomach revealing an obvious infection. The surgeon asks for culture tubes. Answer the following questions about this case.

62

Chapter **7** **Microbes and the Process of Infection**

116. What equipment and supplies do you request from your circulator?

117. What tests or exams is the surgeon most likely to order for this case?

118. What tests or exams are available from which the surgeon can choose?

119. Which test will the surgeon request if she wants or needs an immediate answer so that she can treat her patient?

INTERNET EXERCISES

Internet Exercise 1

Go online and search for information about the risk factors for a surgical site infection. When you find a site, use it to answer the following questions.

120. How does the patient's age affect the surgical wound if it is originally classified as clean?

121. Why is a malnourished patient more likely to have a wound infection or delayed wound healing?

122. Why would IDDM cause the surgical wound to be at risk for infection?

123. Why would a patient with lupus be at risk for a surgical wound infection?

Internet Exercise 2

Go online to the Web site for the Centers for Disease Control and Prevention (CDC). Find the information to fill in the chart below.

Microbe	Morphology	Disease	Port of entry
Staphylococcus aureus			
Staphylococcus epidermis			
Streptococcus pyogenes			
Pseudomonas aeruginosa			
Neisseria gonorrhoeae			
Neisseria meningitidis			
Bordetella pertussis			
Enteric bacteria			

Microbe	Morphology	Disease	Port of entry
Escherichia coli			
Salmonella			
Clostridium perfringens			
Clostridium tetani			
Mycobacterium tuberculosis			
Rickettsiae			
HIV			
Human papilloma virus			
Prions			
Creutzfeldt-Jakob disease (CJD)			
Aspergillus fumigatus			
Candida albicans			
Pneumocystis carinii			

Decontamination, Disinfection, and Sterilization

Student's Name _____

KEY TERMS

Write the definition for each term.

1. Antisepsis _____
2. Autoclave _____
3. Bactericidal _____
4. Bacteriostatic _____
5. Biofilm _____
6. Biological indicators _____
7. Cavitation _____
8. Central service department _____
9. Chemical monitor _____
10. Chemical sterilization _____
11. –cidal _____
12. Cleaning _____
13. Cobalt 60 radiation _____
14. Contaminate _____
15. Decontamination _____
16. Disinfection _____
17. Detergent _____
18. Enzymatic cleaner _____
19. Ethylene oxide _____
20. Event-related sterility _____
21. Fungicidal _____
22. Germicidal _____
23. Gravity displacement sterilizer _____
24. High-level disinfection _____
25. High-vacuum sterilizer _____
26. Inanimate _____
27. Indicator _____
28. Noncritical item _____
29. Nonwoven _____

30. Medical device _____

31. Peracetic acid _____

32. Personal protective equipment (PPE) _____

33. Prion _____

34. Process challenge monitoring _____

35. Reprocessing _____

36. Reusable _____

37. Sanitation _____

38. Sharps _____

39. Shelf life _____

40. Single-use items _____

41. Spaulding classification system _____

42. Sporicidal _____

43. Sterilization _____

44. Terminal decontamination _____

45. Ultrasonic cleaner _____

46. Virucidal _____

47. Washer-sterilizer/decontaminator _____

SHORT ANSWERS

Provide a short answer for each question or statement.

48. Before surgery begins, the surgical technologist dons _____, gloves, and gown.

49. CS staff must handle extremely _____ equipment arriving directly from the operating room.

50. Central Service staff must appreciate the need for instrument trays to be _____ and ready in time for their scheduled use.

51. The ultrasonic cleaner removes debris from instruments by a process called _____.

52. Before the washer-sterilizer cycle is finished, the instruments are considered _____.

53. After _____, instruments are taken to the clean assembly area for sorting, inspection, and assembly.

54. Items with a lumen should have a small amount of _____ flushed through them immediately before sterilization.

55. List five of the 10 qualities of a wrapping system.

    a.

    b.

    c.

    d.

    e.

MATCHING

Match each term with the correct definition.

56. _____ Provides recommended practices and technical information for U.S. medical professions

57. _____ Accreditation agency for all health care organizations in the United States

58. _____ Professional association for perioperative nurses

59. _____ An organization for which standards are developed with the support of the U.S. Food and Drug Administration

60. _____ Agency of the federal government that provides research and protocols in all areas of public health

61. _____ Organization that oversees compliance with environmental and patient safety regulations

a. AAMI

b. AORN

c. CD (CDC)

d. TJC

TRUE/FALSE

Indicate whether the statement is true or false.

62. The purpose of decontamination, disinfection, and sterilization is to control the spread of disease by reducing the number of microbes and preventing their proliferation on equipment used in patient care.

    _____ True   _____ False

63. Perioperative staff members put on sterilized scrub attire that has been recently laundered at the start of each working day.

    _____ True   _____ False

64. Disinfecting instruments after they have been used reduces the bioburden.

    _____ True   _____ False

65. The role of the surgical technologist in infection control is to implement the specified procedure correctly and safely according to protocol.

    _____ True   _____ False

Chapter **8** **Decontamination, Disinfection, and Sterilization**

66. The increased acceptance of single-use products has created a need for regulations and recommendations concerning reprocessing of these items.

_____ True   _____ False

67. To save money, some institutions reprocess single-use items.

_____ True   _____ False

68. Sterile equipment that has been opened but has not been used on the patient needs to be reprocessed.

_____ True   _____ False

69. Instruments and equipment do not need to be cleaned before decontamination.

_____ True   _____ False

70. Staff members in the decontamination area must wear PPE.

_____ True   _____ False

71. Only instruments that are free of gross debris are processed in the ultrasonic cleaner.

_____ True   _____ False

To better familiarize yourself with the sequence of events in equipment reprocessing, label the picture of the equipment reprocessing cycle.

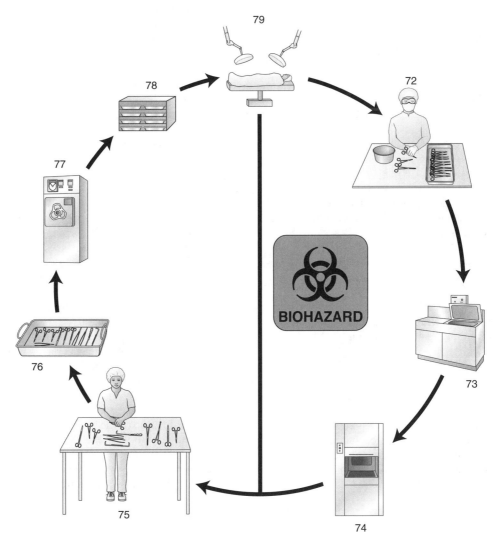

72. _____

73. _____

74. _____

75. _____

76. _____

77. _____

78. _____

79. _____

Choose the most correct answer to complete the question.

80. _____ is a chemical used to remove microorganisms on tissue.
    a. An antiseptic
    b. A disinfectant
    c. Sterilization
    d. All of the above

81. Before and after a surgical case, the floors, walls, and tables are _____ with a detergent.
    a. Cleaned
    b. Processed
    c. Sterilized
    d. Disinfected

82. The system that assigns a device a risk category based on the specific regions of the body where the device is used is the _____ system.
    a. Spaulding
    b. Sterilization
    c. Dewey
    d. Maslow

83. Which of the following body tissues presents a critical risk in the Spaulding system?
    a. Hands
    b. Intact skin
    c. Vascular system
    d. Mucosal membranes

84. _____ is a skilled, certified profession requiring expertise in the science and practice of materials management, decontamination, and sterilization.
    a. Perioperative nursing
    b. Anesthesiology
    c. Central sterile processing
    d. Certified nurse's aides

85. The _____ is used to transport sterile and nonsterile instruments and equipment to and from the main operating room area.
    a. Perioperative nurse
    b. Crash cart
    c. Elevators
    d. Case cart system

86. The washer-sterilizer or washer-disinfector is used to process all instruments that can tolerate
    _____.
    a. Heat
    b. Water turbulence and high-pressure steam
    c. Strong disinfectant
    d. Cold solutions

87. The _____ includes a workroom with ample table space for sorting instruments and assembling instrument sets.
    a. Clean processing area
    b. Decontamination area
    c. Sterile back table
    d. Case cart system

88. Instruments that have _____ must be disassembled before sterilization.
    a. Removable parts
    b. Ratchets
    c. Sharp edges
    d. Blades

89. Instrument trays have a perforated bottom so that:
    a. Steam can circulate up through the tray and adequately cover all surfaces of the instruments.
    b. They are easier for the surgical team to handle.
    c. The instruments are easily put into sets by central processing.
    d. The towels in the instrument sets cannot be damaged by the steam.

90. Which of the following statements is NOT true regarding the use of peel pouches?
    a. Items wrapped in peel pouches must not be placed inside an instrument tray.
    b. Double pouches are unnecessary and may prevent sterilization of the item.
    c. The item in the pouch should clear the seal by at least 1 inch.
    d. Peel pouches are intended for items such as bone rongeurs, rasps, and multiple instruments.

91. Which type of sterilization method requires an aeration time?
    a. Steam
    b. Steam under pressure
    c. Ethylene oxide
    d. Gas plasma

92. Which of the following sterilizers uses peracetic acid?
    a. Steris
    b. Flash
    c. Ethylene oxide
    d. Gas plasma

93. Which of the following high-level disinfectants could also be used as a sterilizing agent?
    a. Gas plasma
    b. Peracetic acid
    c. Glutaraldehyde
    d. Steam

94. _____ is a paper strip or specially treated tape that changes color when exposed to a specific temperature.
    a. Pellet indicator
    b. Chemical monitor
    c. Biological monitor
    d. Air detector

CASE STUDIES

Case Study 1

Read the following case study and answer the following questions.

You are scrubbed into an emergency case involving a patient with a fractured hip. The instruments that your hospital uses to repair the fracture were used earlier in the day and are not sterile. The set includes the implants. You put the instruments in the flash sterilizer, and once scrubbed in and ready, you retrieve them from the autoclave. The case begins without incident.

95. At what temperature did you run the instruments?

_____

96. For how many minutes did you set the autoclave to run?

_____

97. How do you know the instruments have been through the sterilization process when you retrieve them?

_____

_____

98. How do you know the instruments are "most likely" sterile?

_____

_____

Case Study 2

99. In the case study above, you should be concerned about the "process-related parameters" for steam sterilization. What are they?

_____

_____

Chapter **8** Decontamination, Disinfection, and Sterilization

Internet Exercise 1

*Using your favorite search engine, do research using the key words **prion** and **Creutzfeldt-Jakob disease (CJD)**. Then answer the following questions about your research.*

100. What are prions?

_____

_____

101. What causes CJD?

_____

_____

102. Why is CJD a concern with regard to sterilization methods?

_____

_____

9 | Aseptic Technique

KEY TERMS

Write the definition for each term.

1. Airborne contamination _____
2. Antiseptics _____
3. Asepsis _____
4. Aseptic technique _____
5. Centers for Disease Control and Prevention (CDC) _____
6. Chemical barrier _____
7. Closed gloving _____
8. Contamination _____
9. Gross contamination _____
10. Hand washing _____
11. Hand antisepsis _____
12. Latex allergy _____
13. Nonsterile personnel _____
14. Open gloving _____
15. Pathogenic _____
16. Physical barrier _____
17. Resident flora _____
18. Scrub _____
19. Scrubbed personnel _____
20. Sharps _____
21. Standard Precautions _____
22. Sterile field _____
23. Sterile item _____
24. Sterility _____
25. Strike-through contamination _____
26. Surfactant _____
27. Surgical conscience _____

28. Surgical hand rub _____

29. Surgical hand scrub _____

30. Surgical site infection (SSI) _____

31. Topical antiseptics (antimicrobials) _____

32. Transient flora _____

SHORT ANSWERS

Provide a short answer for each question or statement.

33. What are the four methods of aseptic technique?

    a.

    b.

    c.

    d.

34. Minor breaks in aseptic technique usually can be corrected as _____.

35. The methods used to achieve the goal of asepsis are called _____.

36. Items exposed (opened) to the surgical field are considered _____ after they have been exposed to the air or to a patient's tissues.

37. Sterile objects are contained or confined to avoid contact with _____ objects.

38. Body piercing is considered jewelry and ideally should be _____.

39. Describe when a surgical technologist might choose to use a bouffant cap or a surgeon's cap rather than a head cover.

    _____

    _____

    _____

40. The primary purpose of shoe covers is to _____.

41. _____ are the two types of hand hygiene practiced in the operating room and other health care settings.

42. Explain where the surgical gown is considered sterile. _____

_____

_____

MATCHING

Match each term with the correct definition.

43. _____ The application of an approved antiseptic to all surfaces
of the hands and fingers

44. _____ A process meant to reduce the number of microorganisms
on the skin to an absolute minimum

45. _____ A timed surgical scrub

46. _____ Counted strokes

47. _____ Ethyl or isopropyl alcohol combined with skin emollients

48. _____ Should be used only when no soil is visible on the hands

49. _____ Brushes must be sterile

50. _____ Event related

a. Hand washing
b. Hand antisepsis
c. Surgical scrub

TRUE/FALSE

Indicate whether the statement is true or false.

51. Universal Precautions were established to prevent the spread of HIV and AIDS.

_____ True   _____ False

52. The term *sterile* is absolute.

_____ True   _____ False

53. Admitting and reporting any break in technique demonstrates a low level of professional maturity and surgical
conscience.

_____ True   _____ False

54. A physical barrier is one that contains (encloses) or separates a source of contamination.

_____ True   _____ False

55. No evidence indicates that open sores, cuts, or small skin wounds harbor bacteria that are spread in the course of
handling of surgical equipment.

_____ True   _____ False

56. Jewelry of any kind is a potential source of pathogens.

_____ True   _____ False

57. The scrub top should be secured at the waist and tucked into the pants or should fit close to the body to prevent contact with sterile surfaces.

_____ True   _____ False

58. Surgical site infections have been traced to *S. aureus* and group A streptococci.

_____ True   _____ False

59. All surgical team members must wear impervious protective eyewear or face shields during all procedures and whenever the risk exists that blood, body fluids, or particles of tissue could splash on the face.

_____ True   _____ False

60. All practices that prevent the transmission of infectious disease in the health care setting flow from standards called *Standard Precautions*.

_____ True   _____ False

61. When used properly, masks block droplets and filter air.

_____ True   _____ False

MULTIPLE CHOICE

Choose the most correct answer to the question or statement.

62. Which of the following is NOT an example of EBP?
    a. Double gloving
    b. Surgical hand scrub
    c. Surgical hand rub
    d. Patient surgical site scrub

63. After an item has been sterilized, its sterility is maintained by _____.
    a. Surgical technologists
    b. Asepsis
    c. Decontamination
    d. Aseptic technique

64. The ethical and professional motivation that regulates a professional's behavior regarding disease transmission is known as _____.
    a. Tort
    b. Surgical law
    c. Surgical conscience
    d. Asepsis

65. A scrub suit must be changed if it:
    a. Is contaminated by blood or body fluids
    b. Comes in contact with the patient
    c. Comes in contact with any nonsterile item
    d. Leaves the operating room

66. Long-sleeved cover jackets are worn by the _____.
    a. Surgeon
    b. Scrub
    c. Circulator
    d. All of the above

67. At the end of the shift, the surgical technologist may place the scrub suit in his or her locker if:
    a. It is unsoiled.
    b. It does not have gross contaminants on it.
    c. The surgical technologist has worked less than 8 hours in it.
    d. The hospital does not want to launder the scrub suits frequently.

68. When changing from street clothes to a scrub suit for entering the operating room, the surgical technologist puts on which of the following items first?
    a. Scrub pants
    b. Shoe covers
    c. Scrub shirt
    d. Head covering

69. The term for the area under the fingernails is _____.
    a. Sublingual
    b. Subungual
    c. Buccal
    d. Unguintine

70. In the surgical scrub, which of the following comes first?
    a. Scrubbing the forearms
    b. Scrubbing the fingers
    c. Scrubbing the nail beds
    d. Applying the soap from fingers to elbows to "wash" the hands and arms

71. The surgical scrub extends to:
    a. 2 inches above the elbows
    b. The elbows
    c. Just below the elbows
    d. The shoulders

72. When sterile supplies have been opened, the sterile setup is vulnerable to contamination. As a surgical technologist, you recognize that once the sterile supplies have been opened, you:
    a. Have no further obligation to the items
    b. Know that the items are safe from contamination if you shut the OR door
    c. Know that you must ask a nurse's aide to stand at the closed door
    d. Must constantly monitor the sterile supplies

73. No data currently are available to suggest that leaving a sterile setup exposed increases the risk of _____.
    a. Patient death
    b. Surgical site infections
    c. Contamination
    d. Complications

74. _____ is a way of making decisions and acting on proven methods.
    a. Evidence-based practice
    b. Surgical conscience
    c. Asepsis
    d. Aseptic technique

CASE STUDIES

Case Study 1

Read the following case study and answer the questions about opening a sterile table.

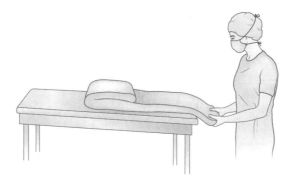

Look at the preceding picture and answer the following questions about the actions of the surgical technologist.

Chapter **9** **Aseptic Technique**

The surgical technologist has just opened one side of her sterile table. What are her next three actions? (Be specific.)

75. _____

76. _____

77. _____

Case Study 2

You are a certified surgical technologist (CST), and you have been assigned to discuss aseptic technique with a group of nursing students. You will want to discuss each of the 16 areas discussed in the text and give an example of each. What are they?

78. _____

79. _____

80. _____

81. _____

82. _____

83. _____

84. _____

85. _____

86. _____

87. _____

88. _____

89. _____

90. _____

91. _____

92. _____

93. _____

Internet Exercise 1

Go online to the Web site for the Centers for Disease Control and Prevention (CDC). See whether you can find the two organisms listed in your text as causative agents for a surgical site infection (SSI). Using the Web site, answer the following questions about your research.

94. What Web site did you use? Give the Web site "address" (URL).

_____

95. What organisms did you research?

_____

96. Where are these organisms in their normal habitat?

_____

97. Did you find other organisms that are common flora for humans? If so, list them.

_____

10 Transporting, Transferring, and Positioning the Surgical Patient

Student's Name _____

KEY TERMS

Write the definition for each term.

1. Abduction _____

2. Compartment syndrome _____

3. Compression injury _____

4. Dependent area of the body _____

5. Embolism _____

6. Fasciotomy _____

7. Fowler's position _____

8. Hyperextension _____

9. Hyperflexion _____

10. Hypotension _____

11. Ischemia _____

12. Jackknife or Kraske's position _____

13. Knee-chest position _____

14. Lateral position _____

15. Lithotomy position _____

16. Log roll _____

17. Necrosis _____

18. Neuropathy _____

19. Prone position _____

20. Range of motion _____

21. Reverse Trendelenburg position _____

22. Semi-Fowler position _____

23. Shear injury _____

24. Supine position _____

25. Table break _____

26. Thoracic outlet syndrome _____

27. Thromboembolus _____

28. Traction injury _____

29. Transfer board _____

30. Trendelenburg's position _____

31. Ventilation _____

SHORT ANSWERS

Provide a short answer for each question or statement.

32. What is a transfer board used for? _____

33. What type of activity would or could cause a shearing injury? _____

34. What did the author mean when she wrote in the text that "positioning the surgical patient is not a cookbook activity"?

_____

_____

35. Why are health care workers at high risk for back injury and musculoskeletal injury while moving and transferring patients?

_____

_____

_____

36. List three risk factors for patient injury when patients are transported or transferred:

a.

b.

c.

37. What are the three ways that all health care workers should identify the patient?

1.

2.

3.

38. What are the steps taken to transfer a patient from a bed to a wheelchair?

_____

_____

39. What are the steps taken to assist a patient in moving from a lying position to a sitting position?

_____

_____

40. Name the three elements of safe positioning of a patient.

a.

b.

c.

LABELING

Label the operating room table in the following figure.

41. (1) _____

42. (2) _____

43. (3) _____

44. (4) _____

45. (5) _____

46. (6) _____

47. (7) _____

48. (8) _____

49. (9) _____

50. (10) _____

51. (11) _____

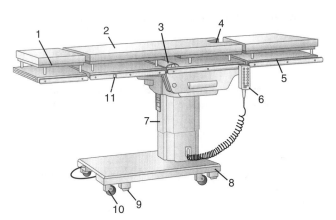

Modified from Martin JT, Warner MA: *Positioning in anesthesia and surgery,* ed 3, Philadelphia, 1997, WB Saunders.

MATCHING

Match each term with the correct definition. Some terms may be used more than once.

52. _____ Position in which the patient's head is tilted down

53. _____ Position in which the patient is lying on the back

54. _____ Sitting position

55. _____ Position in which the patient's feet are tilted down

56. _____ Position in which the patient is lying with the front of the body (the abdomen) on the operating room table

57. _____ Position used for vaginal, perineal, and rectal procedures

58. _____ Position used for neck and thyroid procedures

59. _____ A type of prone position in which the patient's hips are flexed in an inverted V

60. _____ Sitting position used for cranial, facial, and reconstructive breast procedures

61. _____ Side-lying position

62. _____ Semisitting position

a. Semi-Fowler position

b. Reverse Trendelenburg position

c. Prone position

d. Lithotomy position

e. Trendelenburg's position

f. Supine position

g. Jackknife (Kraske's) position

h. Lateral position

i. Fowler's position

Chapter **10** **Transporting, Transferring, and Positioning the Surgical Patient**

Indicate whether the statement is true or false.

63. Health care workers are at high risk for back injury and other types of musculoskeletal injury while caring for, moving, and transferring patients.

_____ True _____ False

64. Many patients fear that their personal rights, such as a right to modesty, are forfeited upon admission to the hospital.

_____ True _____ False

65. All patients are identified in at least two different ways.

_____ True _____ False

66. If the patient's name, hospital identification number, surgery, and surgical site do not match the chart or operative documents, you must report this to the unit charge nurse.

_____ True _____ False

67. When a patient is transferred from a bed to a stretcher or wheelchair, the equipment is transferred first and then the patient.

_____ True _____ False

68. Before transporting the patient, you should notify the unit clerk that you have arrived to transport the patient to surgery.

_____ True _____ False

69. When transporting the patient by stretcher, you should stand at the patient's head and push the stretcher forward, feet first.

_____ True _____ False

70. It is permissible to transport the patient in an elevator full of family and visitors.

_____ True _____ False

71. The surgical technologist is allowed to receive the patient into the operating room if the circulator and anesthesiologist are busy or not present.

_____ True _____ False

72. There is only one correct way to move a patient from the stretcher to the operating room table, and that is a patient roller.

_____ True _____ False

Choose the most correct answer to complete the question or statement.

73. Which of the following terms means movement of a joint or body part away from the body?
    a. Abduction
    b. Adduction
    c. Hyperextension
    d. Ischemia

74. Health care workers are at high risk for injury while caring for, moving, and transferring patients because:
    a. They do not use proper body mechanics when moving a patient.
    b. The tasks are unpredictable.
    c. A sudden shift of the patient's weight may put the worker off balance.
    d. All of the above.

75. Transport and transfer injuries occur more often when:
    a. There is sufficient help.
    b. Personnel assisting in the transfer or transport have a plan.
    c. Personnel are rushed.
    d. The patient is cooperative.

76. Which of the following statements is true regarding patient transfers?
    a. One person should be in charge of the move and guide the others.
    b. It is best to make a plan as you move the patient so that the move is individualized.
    c. The patient's right to modesty is forfeited at admission.
    d. It is best to move the patient without blankets so that the patient does not get tangled up in them.

77. The most important part of transporting patients is _____.
    a. Proper identification before you transport them
    b. Proper positioning on the cart
    c. Keeping the patient warm while in the hallways
    d. Greeting the patient in a friendly manner and introducing yourself

78. The first step in transferring a mobile patient to a stretcher is to:
    a. Lower the bed rails and align the patient's bed and the stretcher
    b. Make sure the locks are engaged on both the patient's bed and the stretcher
    c. Identify the patient
    d. Let the surgeon know that the patient is about to be transferred

79. _____ people should be present during the transfer of a mobile and alert patient.
    a. Two or three
    b. Three or four
    c. Four or five
    d. Five or six

80. The transfer of a conscious patient from a stretcher to an operating table starts with aligning the head of the stretcher with the head of the operating table and then:
    a. Opening up the back of the patient's gown
    b. Identifying the patient
    c. Freeing up the IV tubing
    d. Locking the wheels of the stretcher and the operating room table

81. During the transfer of a conscious patient to the operating room table, the duties of the anesthesiologist include:
    a. Protecting the patient's neck and airway
    b. Holding the IV tubing
    c. Controlling the slide board
    d. Nothing; the anesthesiologist does not assist in the move

CASE STUDIES

Case Study 1

Read the following case study and answer the questions based on your knowledge of patient positioning and use of the operating room table.

You have been asked to set up the operating room for a procedure. Today your surgeon will perform an open thoracotomy in operating room 2. The surgeon has told the team that he will be making an incision in the right intercostal area.

82. In what position will the patient be placed? _____

83. The patient will be in what position for administration of the general anesthetic?

_____

84. What positioning devices will be needed for this patient? _____

_____

_____

INTERNET EXERCISES

Internet Exercise 1

*Using your favorite search engine, go online and search for the key words **surgical positioning** and **neuropathy**. Then answer the following questions.*

85. What did you find in your search that surprised you or that you did not already know about how patients can suffer from improper positioning in the operating room?

_____

_____

_____

Internet Exercise 2

*Using your favorite search engine, go online and search for the key words **brachial plexus**. Then answer the following questions.*

86. What is the brachial plexus? _____

_____

87. Where is the brachial plexus? _____

_____

88. What nerves are involved with the structure? _____

_____

89. How is the brachial plexus injured? _____

_____

11 Surgical Skin Preparation and Draping

Student's Name _____

Write the definition for each term.

1. Antiseptic _____

2. Barrier drape _____

3. Debridement _____

4. Decompression _____

5. Desiccation _____

6. Drape _____

7. Fenestrated drape _____

8. Head drape _____

9. Impervious _____

10. Incise drapes _____

11. Prep _____

12. Residual activity _____

13. Retention catheter _____

14. Sterile field _____

15. Straight catheter _____

16. Surgical site infection (SSI) _____

In the drawings below, use a colored pen or pencil to indicate the prep for the procedure listed.

17. Anterior head and neck

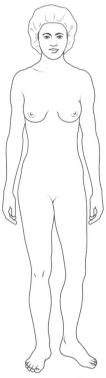

Modified from Phillips N: *Berry and Kohn's operating room technique*, ed 10, 2004, Mosby.

18. Anterior shoulder

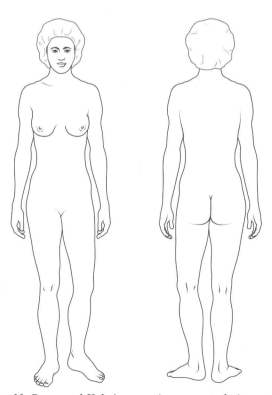

Modified from Phillips N: *Berry and Kohn's operating room technique*, ed 10, 2004, Mosby.

Chapter **11 Surgical Skin Preparation and Draping**

19. Back

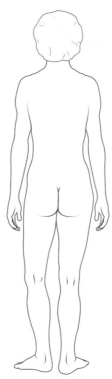

Modified from Phillips N: *Berry and Kohn's operating room technique*, ed 10, 2004, Mosby.

20. Abdomen

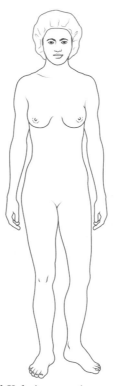

Modified from Phillips N: *Berry and Kohn's operating room technique*, ed 10, 2004, Mosby.

21. Inguinal area

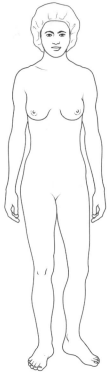

Modified from Phillips N: *Berry and Kohn's operating room technique*, ed 10, 2004, Mosby.

SHORT ANSWERS

Provide a short answer for each question or statement.

22. Urinary catheterization is necessary in selected procedures and circumstances. What are they?

    a.

    b.

    c.

    d.

23. What are the risks involved in improper use of prep solutions?

    a.

    b.

    c.

24. Why is iodine a risk of chemical burn when it is heated (warmed)? _____

_____

92

25. What measures are taken to ensure that the correct site is prepped? _____

_____

_____

26. What guidelines should be followed for hair removal?

 a.

 b.

 c.

 d.

 e.

 f.

 g.

 h.

 i.

27. The flank and back areas are prepped in the same manner as the abdomen; describe the technique here.

_____

_____

_____

28. What is the purpose of surgical draping? _____

_____

29. Before starting the skin prep, the surgical technologist should perform a mental check of patient safety considerations. This includes:

 a.

 b.

 c.

MATCHING

Match each term with the correct definition. Some terms may be used more than once.

30. _____ Retains its microbicidal action in the presence of organic substances

31. _____ Destroys microorganisms through desiccation

32. _____ Provides residual activity

33. _____ Has limited use in surgery; is nontoxic and can be used in the area of the eyes and ears

34. _____ Has been linked to hearing loss when accidentally introduced into the middle ear

35. _____ Commonly found in deodorants, antibacterial soaps, and other proprietary cosmetics

36. _____ Not effective in the presence of soap and organic debris such as skin oils, blood, and body fluids

37. _____ Absorbed through the skin and may cause toxicity

38. _____ Extremely flammable and volatile

a. Alcohol

b. Chlorhexidine gluconate (CHG)

c. Iodophors

d. Triclosan

e. Parachlorometaxylenol

TRUE/FALSE

Indicate whether the statement is true or false.

39. Before surgery, the skin must be cleansed with disinfectants to sterilize it.

_____ True   _____ False

40. Skin prep begins before the patient arrives in surgery.

_____ True   _____ False

41. Patients wear clean hospital attire because it contributes to overall asepsis.

_____ True   _____ False

42. Catheterization often is performed immediately before the surgical skin prep.

_____ True   _____ False

43. The patient's allergy status must be verified before insertion of a Foley catheter.

_____ True   _____ False

44. During insertion of a Foley catheter, if the insertion hand becomes contaminated, the procedure must be stopped and the contaminated glove changed.

_____ True   _____ False

45. If at any time during urinary catheter insertion blood returns through the urethra, the procedure should be completed quickly before further complications arise.

_____ True   _____ False

46. Urinary catheterization is the most common cause of hospital-acquired infections in the United States.

_____ True   _____ False

47. The skin is the body's primary defense against infection.

_____ True   _____ False

48. Only antiseptic agents approved for use on the skin may be used for the prep.

_____ True   _____ False

MULTIPLE CHOICE

Choose the most correct answer to complete the question or statement.

49. The patient is ready for skin prep and draping only after _____.
   a. induction of general anesthesia and intubation
   b. the "pause"
   c. the circulator has finished the required surgical paperwork
   d. the surgeon inspects the patient's surgical site skin

50. A retention catheter with a small, inflatable balloon at the tip is called a _____ catheter.
   a. Robinson
   b. Malcot
   c. Fogarty
   d. Foley

51. Selection of the correct catheter is based on the patient's:
   a. Age, mental development, and sexual preference
   b. Age, size, and the type of procedure
   c. Age, size, and gender
   d. Size, grade in school, and gender

52. Catheterization of a female surgical patient requires the _____ position.
   a. Supine
   b. Prone
   c. Lithotomy
   d. Knees slightly flexed

53. Which of the following statements is true regarding the technique for placing a Foley catheter?
   a. The assisting hand does not contact sterile supplies, including the catheter itself.
   b. Both hands must remain sterile for the procedure.
   c. If the catheter is placed before the prep has been done, it is not done using aseptic technique.
   d. The insertion hand does not contact sterile supplies.

54. Skin is naturally _____.
   a. Sterile
   b. Bacteria free
   c. Greasy
   d. Water repellant

55. When is hair removed from the surgical site?
   a. When it is ordered by the surgeon
   b. If it will interfere with the procedure
   c. When the patient has excess hair
   d. When the patient is a high risk for surgical site infection

56. Which of the following is NOT true regarding the two methods of prepping?
   a. Antiseptic soap solution is used, followed by a coating of antiseptic.
   b. Antiseptic solution alone is used.
   c. The prep used is based on the surgeon's orders.
   d. The prep used is based on the preferences of the hospital infection control nurse.

57. The basic principles of the skin prep _____.
   a. Vary from patient to patient
   b. Are based on the rules of aseptic technique
   c. Vary from procedure to procedure
   d. Are based on hospital policy and surgeon's preference

58. Surgeons apply the surgical drapes in a prescribed order based on _____.
   a. Aseptic technique
   b. Surgical practice
   c. The patient's risk of infection
   d. Hospital policy

59. To ensure a moisture barrier between the patient and the sterile field, surgical drapes are made of woven and _____ materials.
   a. Polypropylene
   b. Linen
   c. Bonded synthetic
   d. Polyester

60. A draping routine usually begins with _____.
   a. A plain sheet of some type
   b. A stockinette
   c. A fenestrated drape
   d. A towel or sticky drape

61. The sterile drape that is coated with adhesive on one side and may be impregnated with antiseptic is called a (an) _____.
   a. Three-quarter drape
   b. Fenestrated drape
   c. Half-sheet
   d. Incise drape

62. The procedure drape or specialty drape is placed on the patient _____.
   a. Before the half-sheet
   b. Before the incise drape
   c. First
   d. Last

63. Which of the following rules of asepsis apply to placement of the surgical drapes?
   a. Handle drapes with as much movement as you need to ensure proper placement.
   b. When placing a drape, do not touch the patient's body.
   c. After a drape has been placed, shift or move the drape to make a good fit for the patient and the procedure.
   d. Use towel clamps to secure drapes.

64. The sterile technique required for catheterization entails keeping _____.
   a. Both hands and arms sterile
   b. Both hands unsterile, because this is not a sterile procedure
   c. One hand sterile and the other hand nonsterile
   d. Both hands sterile

CASE STUDIES

Case Study 1

Read the following case study and answer the questions based on your knowledge of insertion of a urinary catheter.

Your surgical patient has been released to you for prepping and draping by the anesthesia provider. The surgeon has requested placement of a Foley catheter for this procedure.

65. Before you begin the procedure, you check the patient's chart for allergies. Why is this particularly important for placement of a Foley catheter?

_____

_____

_____

66. What is the job of the "assisting hand" during insertion of a urinary catheter?

_____

_____

_____

67. What is the job of the "insertion hand" during urinary catheter insertion?

_____

_____

_____

Case Study 2

Read the following case study and answer the questions based on your knowledge of surgical drapes.

You are about to scrub for a knee arthroscopy. Your patient is asleep under general anesthesia. He has been prepped, and you are about to drape him. What will you need to have ready for the surgeon so that you can drape the patient? List your supplies in the order you will use them.

68. _____

69. _____

70. _____

71. _____

INTERNET EXERCISES

Internet Exercise 1

Using your favorite search engine, type in the key words and/or abbreviations **SSI, urinary site infections,** *and* **nosocomial infections.** *Answer the following questions about your research.*

72. What did you find out about the incidence of SSIs and urinary infections?

_____

_____

73. When you looked up nosocomial infection, how many times did urinary site infections come up?

_____

_____

74. Did you find statistics indicating the percentage of surgical or hospital infections related to catheter placement?

_____

_____

12 Anesthesia, Anesthetics, and Physiological Monitoring

Student's Name _____

KEY TERMS

Write the definition for each term.

1. Airway _____

2. Amnesia _____

3. Analgesia _____

4. Anaphylaxis _____

5. Anesthesia care provider (ACP) _____

6. Anesthesia machine _____

7. Anesthesia technician _____

8. Anesthesiologist _____

9. Anesthetic _____

10. Antagonist _____

11. Antegrade amnesia _____

12. Anxiolytic _____

13. Apnea _____

14. Bispectral index system _____

15. Bolus injection _____

16. Breathing bag _____

17. Bronchospasm _____

18. CRNA _____

19. Coma _____

20. Controlled hypothermia _____

21. Cricoid pressure _____

22. Cyanosis _____

23. Delirium _____

24. Emergence _____

25. Endotracheal tube _____

26. Esmarch bandage _____

27. Extubation _____

28. Gas scavenging _____

29. Homeostasis _____

30. Hypertonic _____

31. Hypothermia _____

32. Hypotonic _____

33. Induction _____

34. Infusion _____

35. Intraoperative awareness _____

36. Intubation _____

37. Isotonic _____

38. Laryngeal mask airway (LMA) _____

39. Laryngoscope _____

40. Malignant hyperthermia _____

41. Monitored anesthesia care _____

42. Neuromuscular blocking agent _____

43. Pneumatic tourniquet _____

44. Postanesthesia recovery unit (PACU) _____

45. Protective reflexes _____

46. Pulse oximeter _____

47. Perfusion _____

48. Regional block _____

49. Sedative _____

50. Sensation _____

51. Unconsciousness _____

52. Ventilation _____

SHORT ANSWERS

Provide a short answer for each question or statement.

53. What are the five senses?

    a.

    b.

    c.

    d.

    e.

54. Besides the "five senses," the nervous system is capable of other sensations. What are they?

    _____

    _____

55. List three of the responsibilities of the ACP.

a.

b.

c.

56. What six things help the surgeon, the ACP, and the patient decide which type of anesthetic will be best for the individual during the procedure?

a.

b.

c.

d.

e.

f.

57. Hospitals and other surgical facilities have individual check-in protocols. Which specific details are always verified?

a.

b.

c.

d.

e.

f.

g.

h.

i.

58. General anesthesia is the reversible loss of consciousness, which is accompanied by the absence of:

a.

b.

c.

d.

e.

f.

59. What are the four phases of anesthesia?

a.

b.

c.

d.

60. Describe the types of conscious sedation. _____

_____

_____

LABELING

Name the instrument shown in each figure.

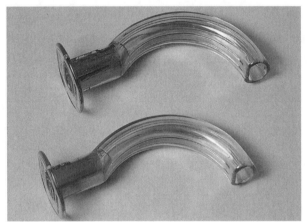

From Elkin MK, Perry PA: *Nursing interventions and clinical skills*, ed 4, St Louis, 2007, Mosby.

61. _____

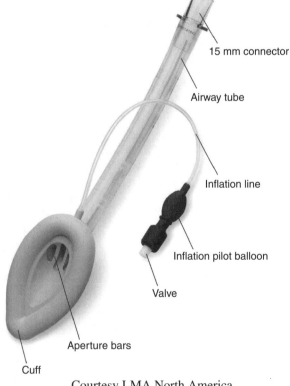

15 mm connector

Airway tube

Inflation line

Inflation pilot balloon

Valve

Aperture bars

Cuff

Courtesy LMA North America.

62. _____

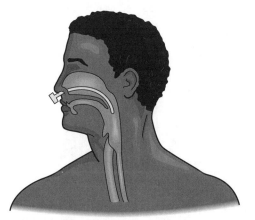

Modified from Sorrentino SA: *Mosby's textbook for nursing assistants,* ed 5, St Louis, 2000, Mosby.

63. _____

Modified from Sorrentino SA: *Mosby's textbook for nursing assistants,* ed 5, St Louis, 2000, Mosby.

64. _____

CHART COMPLETION

Using your knowledge of the drugs used for general anesthesia and conscious sedation, fill in the following chart. An example is given for you.

Name	Drug classification	Advantages and uses	Disadvantages
Example: Nitrous oxide	*Inhalation agent*	*Decreased incidence of nausea and rapid absorption and clearance from the body*	*Low potency and lack of muscle relaxation*
65. Isoflurane			
66. Sevoflurane			
67. Desflurane			
68. Halothane/ Ethrane			
69. Propofol			
70. Etomidate			
71. Thiopental			
72. Ketamine			
73. Benzodiazepines			
74. Succinylcholine			

Chapter **12** **Anesthesia, Anesthetics, and Physiological Monitoring**

75. Mivacurium			
76. Neostigmine			
77. Morphine sulfate 　　Meperidine 　　Alfentanil 　　Fentanyl 　　Sufentanil			
78. Narcan 　　Naloxone			
79. Atropine sulfate			
80. Scopolamine			

MATCHING

Match each term with the correct definition.

81. _____ Without sensation

82. _____ Anesthesia in which the agent is injected into a vein

83. _____ The use of multiple drugs to produce sedation, analgesia, amnesia, and muscle relaxation

84. _____ Associated with a state of unconsciousness

85. _____ Anesthesia in a specific area of the body induced by injection of the anesthetic around a major nerve or group of nerves

86. _____ Anesthesia of superficial nerves

87. _____ The monitoring of vital functions during regional anesthesia

a. Bier block

b. Topical anesthesia

c. Monitored anesthesia care

d. General anesthesia

e. Balanced anesthesia

f. Anesthesia

g. Regional block

TRUE/FALSE

Indicate whether the statement is true or false.

88. The goal of surgical anesthesia is to allow the patient to tolerate surgery and maintain the body in a balanced physiological state called *homeostasis*.

_____ True　　　　　_____ False

89. Modern anesthesia is characterized by an alteration in the patient's sensory awareness and consciousness.

_____ True　　　　　_____ False

90. In a fully conscious person, some of the autonomic and sensory functions are intact and the patient is "awake."

_____ True　　　　　_____ False

91. "Central nervous system depression" is another term for sedation.

_____ True   _____ False

92. Chemicals that carry impulses from nerve cell to nerve cell are called *neurotransmitters*.

_____ True   _____ False

93. If a drug potentiates release and/or uptake of a particular neurotransmitter, it is called an *antagonist*.

_____ True   _____ False

94. Neuromuscular blocking agents are used during surgery to relax or paralyze muscles.

_____ True   _____ False

95. The ACP monitors the patient from the time the patient enters the surgical suite until the patient is discharged from the PACU.

_____ True   _____ False

96. Preoperative fasting is required to minimize aspiration (inhalation) of gastric contents during general anesthesia.

_____ True   _____ False

97. A patient who is high risk for aspiration of stomach contents is given drugs to reduce the pH of gastric secretions and reduce gastric volume.

_____ True   _____ False

98. Level of consciousness is monitored to prevent intraoperative awareness (IOA).

_____ True   _____ False

99. Medical-grade gases include oxygen, nitrogen, air, and nitrous oxide.

_____ True   _____ False

100. Local infiltration is the injection of an anesthetic into superficial tissues to produce a small area of anesthesia.

_____ True   _____ False

Choose the most correct answer to complete the question or statement.

101. When the body is in a balanced physiological state, it is in _____.
   a. Hemostasis
   b. Balanced anesthesia
   c. Homeostasis
   d. Topical anesthesia

102. Deep unconsciousness, such as that achieved during general anesthesia, results in the absence of protective mechanisms such as _____.
   a. Blinking and shivering
   b. Cessation of brain activity
   c. Loss of recall
   d. Diminished mental and physical capacity

103. Which of the following is NOT an example of autonomic responses?
   a. Changes in heartbeats
   b. Release of insulin
   c. Peristalsis
   d. Digestion

104. The _____ is responsible for management of postoperative pain.
   a. Surgeon
   b. ACP
   c. RN
   d. Anesthesia tech

105. Hospitals have individual check-in protocols, which may include all of the following details *except* _____.
   a. Patient identity
   b. Correct surgical site
   c. Consent forms
   d. Religious preference

106. Which of the following is NOT considered part of the preoperative routine?
   a. Preoperative fasting
   b. Sedative medication
   c. Prophylactic antibiotics
   d. Inhalation agents

107. Which of the following is a purpose of preoperative medication?
   a. Increase anxiety
   b. Begin induction
   c. Increase gastric volume
   d. Reduce the amount of general anesthetic used

108. Which of the following describes physiological monitoring in the operating room?
   a. A preoperative assessment of the patient's vital metabolic functions
   b. Monitoring that requires patient assessment for clinical signs, interpretation of these signs, and initiation of the appropriate medical response
   c. Physiological monitoring must be done by the anesthesiologist.
   d. Monitoring is necessary because the trauma of surgery has no effect on normal body functions.

109. Which of the following is NOT considered protective reflexes?
   a. Heartbeat
   b. Gagging
   c. Swallowing
   d. Withdrawal from pain

110. Electrocardiography (ECG) measures the _____.
   a. Heart rate per minute
   b. Electrical activity of the brain
   c. Electrical activity of the heart
   d. Respiratory rate per minute

111. Normal body temperature is _____.
   a. 36° to 37.5° C
   b. 95° to 97° C
   c. 94° to 96° F
   d. 36° to 37.5° F

112. A peripheral nerve block:
   a. Provides anesthesia to a specific area of the body
   b. Involves injection of the anesthetic agent into the nerve
   c. Is enervated by a specific nerve
   d. Is done at the end of the procedure for postoperative pain

113. Which of the following would NOT be needed for a Bier block procedure?
   a. Single bladder tourniquet
   b. Esmarch bandage
   c. IV
   d. Lidocaine

Case Study 1

Read the following case study and answer the questions based on your knowledge of the preoperative assessment by the ACP.

You are going to perform a preoperative history and physical on a friend, classmate, or family member using the document on the following page. You will be putting to good use the communication skills learned in Chapter 6 of the textbook. This case study will work out best if you choose someone you don't know very well. That way, you won't be anticipating the answers. You may find that you need to refer to Chapter 12 of the text while interviewing the person. Take your text with you for the interview, and make sure you sign and date your document.

Case Study 2

The American Society of Anesthesiologists (ASA) has developed an assessment system that classifies patients according to risk for anesthesia-related complications. Using that information, rate the following patients.

114. Your 81-year-old patient comes to the emergency department for acute cholecystitis.

    He is classified as a _____.

115. Your 18-year-old patient comes to the hospital for an EGD. The patient currently has medically controlled asthma and has had the problem for about 10 years. He is

    mildly obese. He is classified as a _____.

116. Your 26-year-old patient has come to the hospital for a scheduled cesarean section for delivery of healthy twin babies. She has no underlying disease and will be

    classified as a _____.

117. Your patient is a 39-year-old woman who has insulin-dependent diabetes. She is completely controlled and has kept her blood glucose within normal range by diet, exercise, and insulin for about 6 years. She is coming to the hospital for a tubal

    ligation. She will be classified as a _____.

INTERNET EXERCISES

Internet Exercise 1

*Using your favorite search engine, research information using key words such as **anesthesia, lawsuits,** and **airway complications.** Once you find several sites, answer the following questions. If you cannot answer them, you may need to keep looking.*

118. Did you find any sites that mentioned the patient's dentures being broken during intubation?

    _____

    _____

A	- Absent	☐
C	- Clear	☐
D	- Decreased	☐
R	- Rales	☐
RH	- Rhonchi	☐
W	- Wheezes	☐
SNN	- See Nurses	
	Notes	☐

Addressograph

P.S.S. VITAL SIGNS BP_____ P _____ R _____ T _____ SaO2 _____ (presedative room air)

VITAL SIGNS BP_____ P _____ R _____ T _____ SaO2 _____ (presedative room air)

DATE: _____ TIME: _____

PRE-ANESTHETIC EVALUATION

PRIMARY PHYSICIAN/SURGEON:

PRE-OP DIAGNOSIS:

MEDICATIONS:

CIGARETTES: ☐ QUIT SMOKING _____
ETOH:
DRUG ABUSE: _____

SCHEDULED OPERATION:

REMARKS / FAMILY HEALTH HISTORY:

CARDIOVASCULAR: ☐ ASHD ☐ CHF ☐ H.V.D.
☐ ANGINA ☐ ORTHOPNEA ☐ VALVULAR DISEASE
☐ PREV. M.I. ☐ EDEMA ☐ MVP
☐ ARRHYTHMIA ☐ CYANOSIS ☐ OTHER
☐ THROMBOEMBOLISM ☐ PVD ☐ NEG

RESPIRATORY: ☐ PNEUMONIA ☐ COPD ☐ TRACHEOSTOMY
☐ URI ☐ COUGH ☐ ASTHMA
☐ SOB AT REST ☐ BRONCHITIS ☐ OTHER
☐ SOB W/EXERTION ☐ WHEEZING ☐ NEG

NEUROLOGIC: ☐ SYNCOPE ☐ TIA ☐ LOW BACK PAIN
☐ SEIZURES ☐ COMATOSE ☐ OTHER
☐ CVA ☐ NEUROPATHY ☐ NEG

ENDOCRINE/METABOLIC/RENAL/ HEPATIC: ☐ CIRRHOSIS ☐ DIABETES
☐ ANEMIA ☐ HEPATITIS ☐ HYPOGLYCEMIA
☐ BLEEDING ☐ JAUNDICE ☐ OTHER
☐ SICKLE CELL ☐ CRF ☐ NEG

OTHER: ☐ HIATAL HERNIA ☐ FULL STOMACH ☐ PREGNANCY
☐ H/O MH-FAM ☐ PSYCHIATRIC ☐ NEG

PREVIOUS SURGERIES:
☐ NONE

PREVIOUS ANESTHETIC COMPLICATIONS:
☐ NO KNOWN FAMILY HISTORY OF ANESTHESIA COMPLICATIONS
☐ NONE

REASSESSED IMMEDIATELY PREOP ☐
COMMENTS:

NPO since _____

P.E. AIRWAY MALLAMPATI CLASS 1 2 3 4

ROM: NECK:
TEETH: ☐ DENTURES ☐ CAPS ☐ LOOSE TEETH ☐ CHIPS ☐ RAGGED DENTAL EDGE ☐ PERMANENT BRIDGE
LUNGS:
HEART:
NEURO:

LABS: HGB: _____ ECG ☐ NORMAL
☐ ABNORMAL
HCT: _____ CXR ☐ NORMAL
☐ ABNORMAL
Na+: _____ SMA ☐
K+: _____ CREATININE _____
FBS: _____ PT _____
DOS: _____ PTT _____
PREG TEST: ☐ NEGATIVE
☐ POSITIVE

ASA CLASSIFICATION
1 2 3 4 5 6 E

PROPOSED ANESTHESIA
☐ REGIONAL
☐ IV ☐ EPIDURAL
☐ SPINAL ☐ OTHER
☐ GENERAL
☐ LOCAL W/ SEDATION
☐ LOC/GENERAL
☐ RAPID SEQUENCE INDUCTION

PROPOSED MONITORING
☐ A-LINE
☐ CVP
☐ SWAN

☐ PATIENT CONFUSED, UNABLE TO INTERVIEW
☐ PATIENT RELATIVE INTERVIEWED
☐ RELATIVE UNAVAILABLE
☐ MINOR - MOTHER OR FATHER INTERVIEWED

RISKS/BENEFITS: ☐ DISCUSSED AND UNDERSTOOD
☐ ALL QUESTIONS ANSWERED

SIGNATURE _____

Courtesy St. Joseph's Mercy, Macomb Clinton Township, Mich.

119. Cite one lawsuit that you found.

_____

_____

120. What was the foundation of the lawsuit?

_____

_____

121. What was the amount of damages cited? _____

122. Search for a "policy" regarding the removal of oral piercings and the removal of piercings during general anesthesia. What does the policy state?

_____

_____

123. What Internet site or sites did you use?

_____

_____

_____

13 Postoperative Recovery and Patient Discharge

Student's Name _____

KEY TERMS

Write the definition for each term.

1. Activities of daily living (ADLs) _____

   _____

2. Arterial blood gases (ABGs) _____

   _____

3. Aspiration _____

4. Auscultation _____

5. Bronchospasm _____

6. Discharge against medical advice _____

   _____

7. Discharge criteria _____

   _____

8. Focused assessment _____

   _____

9. Glasgow Coma Scale _____

   _____

10. Handover (hand off) _____

    _____

11. Head to toe assessment _____

12. Hypothermia _____

13. Hypoventilation _____

14. Hypoxia _____

15. Ileus _____

16. Laryngospasm _____

17. Malignant hypothermia _____

18. Perfusion _____

Provide a short answer for each question or statement.

19. List the verbal and written information provided in a handover.

    a.

    b.

    c.

    d.

    e.

    f.

    g.

    h.

20. Why does the perioperative nurse need to report blood loss to the PACU?

    _____

    _____

    _____

    _____

21. During a focused patient assessment in PACU, which specific patient criteria are assessed?

    _____

    _____

22. What is the Glasgow Coma Scale (GSC) and how is it used in the PACU?

    _____

    _____

23. What areas are assessed with the Glasgow Coma Scale?

    _____

    _____

24. Discharge planning and implementation follow established roles and tasks. List them.

(1) _____

(2) _____

(3) _____

(4) _____

(5) _____

(6) _____

MATCHING

Match each term related to postoperative complications with the correct definition.

25. _____ Postoperative nausea and vomiting

26. _____ A rare disease resulting in extremely high core body temperature

27. _____ A blockage of a pulmonary vessel by air, blood clot, or other substance

28. _____ A lack of oxygen to lung tissue

29. _____ Deep vein thrombosis

30. _____ Low blood pressure

31. _____ A sudden collapse of the lung

32. _____ A partial or complete closure of the bronchial tubes

33. _____ Contraction of the laryngeal muscles

a. Hypotension

b. Malignant hyperthermia

c. Anoxia

d. Bronchospasm

e. DVT

f. Pulmonary embolism

g. PONV

h. Atelectasis

i. Laryngospasm

TRUE/FALSE

Indicate whether the statement is true or false.

34. After surgery, patients are transported to the postanesthesia care unit (PACU) for recovery.

_____ True   _____ False

35. Postoperative patients are at risk for complications that may require an emergency medical response.

_____ True   _____ False

36. The PACU is close to the surgical floor (the patient's room) for rapid transfer after surgery.

_____ True   _____ False

37. PACU staff members maintain contact with the family during the intraoperative period.

_____ True   _____ False

38. A brief patient history is relevant to proper assessment of current signs and symptoms and for continuity of nursing care.

_____ True   _____ False

39. Drugs given during the preoperative and intraoperative phases have no effect on drugs administered postoperatively.

_____ True   _____ False

40. Postanesthesia complications occur because patients are physiologically unstable during the immediate postoperative period.

_____ True   _____ False

41. Comfort measures are not important for patients in the PACU, because they are not fully awake yet.

_____ True   _____ False

42. Pain is a complex response to body injury and is affected by previous experience.

_____ True   _____ False

43. Before discharge from PACU, the patient must be able to perform activities of daily living with some degree of independence or have help in dressing, eating, mobilizing, and toileting.

_____ True   _____ False

MULTIPLE CHOICE

Choose the most correct answer to complete the question or statement.

44. In a handover, the circulator is essentially:
    a. Sending the patient to PACU with the transport team
    b. Giving a report on the patient's status to the PACU team
    c. Giving the patient's chart to the floor nurse
    d. Sending a report out to the patient's family during the procedure to keep them informed of the patient's status

45. The patient history includes all of the following *except* _____.
    a. Age
    b. Allergies
    c. Current medications
    d. Future pathology

46. Changes in wound drainage may indicate _____, which requires an immediate medical and nursing response.
    a. Infection
    b. Bleeding
    c. Bruising
    d. None of the above
    e. Both A and B

47. After receiving the handover, the PACU nurse performs a patient _____.
    a. Head to toe assessment
    b. Pain assessment
    c. Social assessment
    d. Wound assessment

48. When assessing the patient's airway, the PACU nurse assesses for _____.
    a. Obstruction, rate, and rhythm
    b. Percussion and obstruction
    c. Breathing and rate
    d. Percussion of the lungs and rate

49. The oxygen saturation of blood is called
   _____.
   a. Hemodynamics
   b. Percussion
   c. Perfusion
   d. Hypoxia

50. Bowel sounds are assessed by _____.
   a. Observation
   b. Palpation
   c. X-ray
   d. Auscultation

51. Assessment for dehydration includes
   _____.
   a. Cardiac dysrhythmia
   b. Alteration in consciousness
   c. Physical signs and symptoms
   d. Blood tests

52. Which of the following are NOT considered
   postoperative complications?
   a. Hypoventilation
   b. Laryngospasm
   c. Coughing
   d. Hypertension

53. Before the patient is discharged from the PACU, the
   staff collaborates with the anesthesia care provider
   and the surgeon to determine whether:
   a. The patient will be safe.
   b. The family has been notified.
   c. The surgeon has had a chance to discuss the
      procedure with the patient.
   d. The anesthesia care provider has approved the
      discharge.

54. Patients are discharged from the PACU only when
   they _____.
   a. Meet discharge criteria
   b. Meet the respiratory standards
   c. Achieve PACU standards
   d. Become normotensive

55. Your surgical patient is about to be discharged from
   PACU. Which of the following does NOT meet the
   criteria for discharge?
   a. The patient arranged for transportation before he
      was admitted for the procedure.
   b. The PACU has called a cab to deliver the patient
      to his apartment.
   c. The patient has asked his friend to assist him to
      his home.
   d. The patient's mother has arrived to drive him
      home and stay with him for the day.

56. It is the responsibility of _____ to
   educate the patient before the individual is
   discharged from the hospital to go home.
   a. Surgical technologist
   b. Surgeon
   c. Anesthesia care provider
   d. Any trained nursing personnel

57. Physiological objectives that are necessary to
   ensure patient safety outside the critical care unit
   are called _____.
   a. APGAR score
   b. Aldrete scale
   c. Discharge planning
   d. Vital signs

58. Pain medications are administered according to all
   of the following *except* _____.
   a. The patient's level of consciousness
   b. The patient's cardiopulmonary status
   c. The patient's age
   d. The patient's mental status

59. The color of the patient's skin and mucous
   membranes may indicate _____.
   a. Hypoxia
   b. Hyperthermia
   c. Hyperoxygenation
   d. Hypovolemia

Case Study 1

Read the following case study and follow the instructions based on your knowledge of the PACU.

You are talking to a friend who is considering a surgical procedure. She asks you about the recovery unit, and you proceed to tell her how the room is arranged. She asks if you could draw a picture for her. Using your text as a guide, draw in the specific details of the PACU.

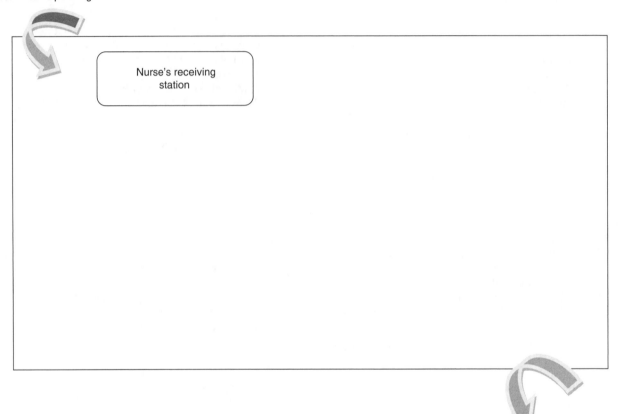

From Main Operating Rooms

Nurse's receiving station

To inpatient rooms

Case Study 2

You are working in the PACU today. Your patient is an 81-year-old man who is IDDM and has just undergone a laparoscopic cholecystectomy for cholelithiasis. You have been asked to see whether he meets the discharge criteria by asking him questions and charting his responses. Each criterion is listed on the following chart. Formulate a question that is appropriate for your PACU patient and then assess whether his response meets the criterion.

• You may need to consult your text to review the criteria.

• Don't forget to use good communication skills for questioning patients. You may need to refer to your text and to Chapter 6 for communication skills.

Discharge criteria	Question	Have criteria been met?
Vital signs		
N&V		
Mobility		
Urinary		
Skin color		
Incision site		
Oriented		
Pain control		
Drinks fluids		
Discharge orders		
Transportation		
Escort		
Home care		
Home environment		

14 Perioperative Pharmacology

Student's Name _____

KEY TERMS

Write the definition for each term.

1. Adverse reaction _____

2. Agonist _____

3. Allergy _____

4. Antagonist _____

5. Antibiotic _____

6. Anticoagulant _____

7. Chemical name _____

8. Concentration _____

9. Contrast medium _____

10. Contraindication_____

11. Controlled substances _____

12. Diuresis _____

13. Dosage _____

14. Dose _____

15. Drug _____

16. Drug administration _____

17. Dye _____

18. Five rights of medication _____

19. Generic name _____

20. Half-life _____

21. Hypersensitivity _____

22. Intraosseous injection _____

23. Intrathecal _____

24. Iodinated contrast medium (ICM) _____

25. Neurotransmitter _____

26. Parenteral _____

27. Peak effect _____

28. Pharmacodynamics _____

29. Pharmacokinetics _____

30. Pharmacology _____

31. Prescription _____

32. Proprietary name _____

33. Side effects _____

34. Stain _____

35. Synergistic _____

36. Topical _____

37. Trade name _____

38. Transdermal _____

39. U.S. Pharmacopeia (USP) _____

SHORT ANSWERS

Provide a short answer for each question or statement.

40. Drugs used in modern medicine are derived from a number of sources. Name four of those sources and give an example of each.

   a. _____

   b. _____

   c. _____

   d. _____

41. The Joint Commission (TJC) requires health care organizations to develop policies that agree with state laws regulating who may handle drugs and in what circumstances. What activities must be regulated?

   a. _____

   b. _____

   c. _____

   d. _____

   e. _____

42. List the 16 drug medication routes. _____

   _____

   _____

   _____

   _____

43. List the four different processes involved in pharmacokinetics.

    a.

    b.

    c.

    d.

44. Increasing the amount of drug beyond the therapeutic level results in _____. The range

    between therapeutic amount and _____ is called the _____.

45. List the four types of allergic reactions and explain the differences between them.

    a. _____

    _____

    b. _____

    _____

    c. _____

    _____

    d. _____

    _____

46. What rights do patients have regarding discussion of drug administration?

    a.

    b.

    c.

    d.

    e.

47. If you are scrubbed and you are about to label the medication on your table, what information must be on the

    label? _____

    _____

48. In Roman numerals, give the year in which you will graduate from your surgical technology program.

    _____

Chapter **14 Perioperative Pharmacology**

49. What time is it in military time if the 10:00 PM news has just started? _____

50. What are the three commonly used staining solutions and what are they used for during the intraoperative period?

   a. _____

   b. _____

   c. _____

51. When are topical antibiotics used for wound irrigation? _____

   _____

   _____

52. What is the difference between a staining agent, a dye, and a contrast medium?

   _____

   _____

   _____

   _____

53. What is the difference between colloids and crystalloids? Give an example of each.

   _____

   _____

   Example of a colloid: _____

   Example of a crystal: _____

MATCHING I

Match each term with the correct definition.

54. _____ A substance taken internally for treatment

55. _____ Manmade

56. _____ The book that contains the standards for quality, strength, packaging, safety, and dosage for all drugs

57. _____ The study of drugs

58. _____ A text published by the World Health Organization (WHO)

59. _____ Any agent that interacts with human tissue

60. _____ Drugs that meet the standards set by the USP are published in this text

a. Pharmacology

b. Synthetic

c. Drugs

d. Pharmaceuticals

e. Physicians' Desk Reference

f. American Hospital Formulary Service Drug Information

g. FDA Orange Book

h. Nursing drug handbooks

61. _____ An online directory of all approved drug products in the United States

62. _____ Contains detailed information about most drugs and is updated yearly

63. _____ Contains less complex information that relates directly to patient care

i. U.S. Pharmacopoeia (USP)

j. International Pharmacopoeia

k. U.S. Pharmacopeia–National Formulary

MATCHING II

Match each term with the correct definition. Some terms may be used more than once.

64. _____ Miconazole

65. _____ Developed during the early 1940s

66. _____ Used in the treatment of respiratory tract infections and sexually transmitted diseases

67. _____ Doxycycline

68. _____ Used selectively because it causes adverse reactions

69. _____ A drug group that is bacteriostatic only

70. _____ Azithromycin

71. _____ Ciprofloxacin

72. _____ Gentamicin

73. _____ For oral administration against rickettsiae

74. _____ Classified into groups called *generations*

a. Penicillin

b. Macrolides

c. Cephalosporins

d. Tetracycline

e. Aminoglycosides

f. Sulfonamides

g. Fluoroquinolones

h. Antifungals

TRUE/FALSE

Indicate whether the statement is true or false.

75. A drug is a chemical substance that alters one or more functions in the body.

_____ True   _____ False

76. Healers of all cultures throughout history have used synthetic substances in the treatment of medical and psychological illness.

_____ True   _____ False

77. Many years of research and testing are needed to prepare a drug for FDA approval.

_____ True   _____ False

78. Drugs that have the potential for abuse are scheduled by the DEA.

_____ True   _____ False

79. Schedule III drugs have less potential for abuse than schedule I drugs.

_____ True   _____ False

80. Drugs classified for pregnancy are classified as schedule I, II, III, IV, or V.

_____ True   _____ False

81. The role of the surgical technologist in handling drugs is to serve as an intermediary between two professionals specifically licensed by their state to administer drugs.

_____ True   _____ False

82. The chemical equivalent of a drug is called the *trade name*.

_____ True   _____ False

83. Improper (or no) medication labeling is a violation of standard operating room procedure and poses a risk to the patient.

_____ True   _____ False

84. Administration of a drug that is beyond its expiration date is a drug error.

_____ True   _____ False

85. The insulin syringe is calibrated in insulin units; the calibrations are incorrect for all drugs except insulin.

_____ True   _____ False

86. The circulator may open the glass ampule and hold it upside down so that the surgical technologist can draw up the medication to deliver it to the sterile field.

_____ True   _____ False

87. By law, drugs with the same generic name must have the same chemical composition, regardless of how many companies produce it.

_____ True   _____ False

88. Anticoagulants are used to dissolve blood clots.

_____ True   _____ False

89. The terms *antibiotic* and *antimicrobial* are not the same.

_____ True   _____ False

90. Diuretics stimulate a shift of body fluids to treat cardiac disorders.

_____ True   _____ False

Choose the most correct answer to complete the question or statement.

91. Drugs that enhance uterine contractions are called _____.
    a. Uterotropics
    b. Pitressin
    c. Synthroid
    d. Isoproterenol

92. In the United States, strict controls and standards are maintained for _____.
    a. All agents used in the body
    b. Only drugs
    c. Only artificial implants and medical devices
    d. Wound closure materials
    e. All of the above

93. Drugs that fall in _____ are determined to have no medical use.
    a. Schedule V
    b. Schedules III and IV
    c. Schedule II
    d. Schedule I

94. Drugs that are classified by pregnancy category include _____.
    a. A, Z, and X
    b. A, B, C, and X
    c. Schedules I, II, III, IV, and V
    d. None of the above

95. Most pregnancy category drugs are listed as _____ because it is unknown whether they pose a risk.
    a. Category A
    b. Schedule C
    c. Category D
    d. Schedule V

96. The route of a drug may not identify the drug's final destination. This statement is true of which of the following drugs?
    a. Injectable lidocaine
    b. IM Ancef
    c. Transdermal nitroglycerine
    d. IV heparin sodium

97. Which of the following medications can be administered intravenously?
    a. Gelfoam
    b. Heparin sodium
    c. Thrombin
    d. Bone wax

98. The action of a drug as it is broken down chemically is called _____.
    a. Passive diffusion
    b. Pharmacokinetics
    c. Pharmacodynamics
    d. Digestion

99. With regard to pharmacokinetics, which of the following processes might involve active transport?
    a. Absorption
    b. Distribution
    c. Metabolism
    d. Excretion

100. The _____ is the amount of time it takes for one half of the drug to be cleared from the body.
    a. Peak and trough
    b. Distribution
    c. Half-life
    d. Metabolism

101. Which of the following would be true when discussing a drug allergy?
    a. The drug/reaction elicits an immune system response.
    b. Drug allergies are a known effect that occurs in some patients.
    c. Drug allergies are treated locally and are rarely serious.
    d. Drug allergies always manifest themselves first by presenting with a rash.

102. Which of the following describes a type II drug allergy?
    a. Anaphylactic shock
    b. Hemolytic disease in newborns
    c. Allergy to antibiotics
    d. A positive reaction to the tuberculin skin test

103. The patient's weight is always calculated for _____.
    a. Pediatric patients
    b. Elderly patients
    c. Patients with diabetes
    d. Adolescents

104. Which of the following is NOT absorbed but is excreted through the GI tract?
    a. Lugol's solution
    b. Methylene blue
    c. Barium
    d. Iodinated contrast medium

105. For what purpose are topical hemostatics used intraoperatively?
    a. To control bleeding from a small capillary complex
    b. To control massive hemorrhage
    c. To assist in the closure of the wound
    d. To promote healing and prevent the formation of a seroma

106. Which of the following is categorized as a topical anticoagulant?
    a. Thrombin
    b. Gelfoam
    c. Heparin sodium
    d. Ostene

107. _____ stimulate the responses of the sympathetic system.
    a. Cholinergics
    b. Antiadrenergics
    c. Adrenergics
    d. Anticholinergics

CASE STUDIES

Case Study 1

Read the following case study and answer the questions.

You have been asked to scrub up and open the room for a vascular case. Your circulator is busy finishing a case in another OR. Because you are a good team member, you want to make sure you have all the supplies you will need for the sterile field, as well as all the supplies your circulator will need. The surgeon's preference card asks for the following medications:

- 1 gram Ancef in 1,000 normal saline irrigation

- 5,000 units heparin sodium in 500 IV NaCl

- Hypaque dye 20/20

- 0.25% Lidocaine with 1:200,000 epinephrine

- 1 vial of methylene blue

108. What are your defined responsibilities in delivering the medication to the sterile field?

    _____

    _____

    _____

    _____

    _____

109. The heparin sodium arrives from the pharmacy in a glass ampule. What method will you use to draw up the medication after you have scrubbed in?

_____

_____

_____

_____

_____

Case Study 2

Read the following case study and answer the questions.

Today you are helping in preoperative holding. Your patient, Mr. Smith, has come down, and you are checking his vital signs. He is in preop holding waiting for his knee arthroscopy to begin. Mr. Smith tells you that he suddenly "does not feel very good." You notice that his face and neck are quite red compared to the rest of his body. You know that the RN in preop holding has just started an IV and administered Mr. Smith's preop antibiotic. You have just recorded that Mr. Smith's vital signs are:

Pulse: 102

Respirations: 14

Blood pressure: 140/74

Temperature: 37° C

Oxygen saturation: 97%

110. What signs do you observe that you believe are not normal for this patient?

_____

111. When did the symptoms start? _____

_____

112. What does the patient report? _____

_____

113. What comfort measures could you initiate? _____

_____

114. Whom do you tell about the change in the patient's condition?

_____

Chapter **14** **Perioperative Pharmacology**

Internet Exercise 1

Surgical technologists are responsible for knowing and complying with the laws and regulations governing drug handling in the state where they live. Research the drug practice acts in your state and answer the following questions.

115. What Internet site did you use?

_____

116. What are the specific laws in your state that help define the role of the surgical tech in the delivery or preparation of medications for the surgical field?

_____

_____

_____

Internet Exercise 2

Now go to www.ast.org, the Web page for the Association for Surgical Technologists (AST).

117. Read through the site for a "scope of practice." What does the national organization say about the role of the surgical tech in the delivery or preparation of medications for the surgical field?

_____

_____

_____

118. Are the national association's scope of practice and the state practice act in your state different?

_____

_____

_____

119. If the two are different, how do you, as a CST, determine your scope of practice?

_____

_____

_____

15 Environmental Hazards

Student's Name _____

KEY TERMS

Write the definition for each term.

1. Airborne transmission precautions _____
2. Blood-borne pathogens _____
3. Genetic mutation _____
4. Latex _____
5. Needleless system _____
6. Neutral zone (no-hands) technique _____
7. Occupational exposure _____
8. Oxygen enriched atmosphere (OEA) _____
9. Personal protective equipment _____
10. Postexposure prophylaxis _____
11. Risk _____
12. Sharps _____
13. Smoke plume _____
14. Standard Precautions _____
15. Transmission-based precautions _____
16. Underwriters Laboratories _____

SHORT ANSWERS

Provide a short answer for each question or statement.

17. List some of the human causes of injury.

_____

_____

_____

_____

_____

18. What are the three areas of potential personal injury?

_____

_____

_____

19. Name the common sources of ignition found in the operating room.

a.

b.

c.

d.

e.

f.

g.

20. What percentage of patient fires occurs inside or on the skin surface?

a.

b.

c.

d.

21. If a fire breaks out in the operating room, what three steps should be taken immediately to protect the patient and put out the fire?

a.

b.

c.

22. Explain the characteristics of electricity. _____

_____

_____

_____

_____

23. All personnel must be familiar with chemical labels and know how to interpret them. What specifically are the guidelines for preventing chemical injury in the operating room?

_____

_____

_____

_____

24. Describe the specific practices of Standard Precautions.

• _____

• _____

• _____

25. What is the neutral zone (no hands) technique? _____

_____

_____

_____

26. What is PEP and what does it involve? _____

_____

_____

27. Transmission-based precautions are implemented when a patient is known or suspected to have a highly infectious disease and Standard Precautions are insufficient to prevent transmission to others. These guidelines are in addition to Standard Precautions. What are they?

• _____

• _____

• _____

Chapter **15 Environmental Hazards**

28. Name five methods that can be used to reduce the risk of sharps injuries.

- _____

- _____

- _____

- _____

- _____

29. List four of the seven suggestions for preventing malfunction in equipment.

a. _____

b. _____

c. _____

d. _____

LABELING

Using the following triangle, draw in the three components required for fire. Under each of the three components, make a directory of the items specific to the operating room that fall into that section.

30. **(1)** _____

_____

_____

31. **(2)** _____

_____

_____

32. **(3)** _____

_____

_____

MATCHING

Match each term with the correct definition.

33. _____ Occupational Safety and Health Administration

34. _____ Environmental Protection Agency

35. _____ Centers for Disease Control and Prevention

36. _____ Association for Professionals in Infection Control and Epidemiology

37. _____ Food and Drug Administration

38. _____ A collaborating agency of WHO

39. _____ National Institute for Occupational Safety and Health

40. _____ www.aorn.org

41. _____ Joint Commission

a. AORN

b. APIC

c. CDC

d. ECRI

e. EPA

f. FDA

g. TJC

h. NIOSH

i. OSHA

TRUE/FALSE

Indicate whether the statement is true or false.

42. High-voltage equipment, chemicals, exposure to blood and body fluids, and stress make the operating room an area with arguably the highest potential for accident and injury in the health care setting.

_____ True   _____ False

43. Risk is the statistical probability of a harmful event that might occur in a given population over a stated period.

_____ True   _____ False

44. In the health care setting, taking a risk for one's self does not include jeopardizing the safety of the patient.

_____ True   _____ False

45. Because oxygen is used in conjunction with an anesthetic, it is termed an OEA.

_____ True   _____ False

46. Items that normally would not burn in atmospheric air are highly flammable in the presence of oxygen.

_____ True   _____ False

47. Alcohol skin prep solutions are a common source of fuel in surgical fires.

_____ True   _____ False

48. Patient fires usually can be contained when two of the three elements of the fire have been removed.

_____ True   _____ False

49. Gases such as oxygen, nitrous oxide, argon, and nitrogen are compressed into metal cylinders for medical use.

_____ True   _____ False

50. Ionizing radiation in amounts high enough to cause tissue damage emanates from x-ray machines.

_____ True   _____ False

51. Distance, exposure, and shielding are the components that are controlled to keep surgical technologists safe as they work with ionizing radiation.

_____ True   _____ False

52. The words *flammable* and *inflammable* have the same meaning.

_____ True   _____ False

MULTIPLE CHOICE

Choose the most correct answer to complete the question or statement.

53. Materials and substances that burn are called
    _____.
    a. Flammable
    b. Flame resistant
    c. Flame retardant
    d. Oxygen rich

54. Which of the following statements is true regarding the high fire risk in the operating room?
    a. Oxygen is heavier than air and settles on the floor.
    b. Oxygen is lighter than air and tends to float above the anesthesia machine.
    c. Oxygen may become confined in areas such as the groin and the axilla.
    d. When nitrous oxide decomposes in the presence of heat, oxygen molecules are produced, creating an oxygen-rich environment.

55. An environment that has a concentration of oxygen greater than 21% is called a/an
    _____.
    a. Oxygen-poor atmosphere
    b. Oxygen-enriched atmosphere
    c. Operating room oxygen
    d. Oxidizer

56. Which of the following are considered flammable?
    a. Endotracheal tubes
    b. Surgical drapes
    c. Fibrin glue
    d. Peroxide

57. Which of the following are considered sources of ignition?
    a. Surgical drapes
    b. Laser
    c. Alcohol
    d. Prepping solution

58. During a colonoscopy, the potential for fire is high because of the high concentration of
    _____.
    a. Flammable drapes and equipment
    b. Oxygen
    c. Laser emissions
    d. Methane gas

59. On which of the following would you use a class A fire extinguisher?
    a. Electrical fires
    b. Laser fires
    c. Flammable liquids
    d. Wood, paper, and cloth

Chapter **15** **Environmental Hazards**

60. Class B fire extinguishers are also called
_____ extinguishers.
a. Bromochlorodifluoromethane
b. Carbon dioxide
c. Hydrogen peroxide
d. Water

61. Which of the following acronyms should you
remember if you are trying to put out a fire?
a. PASS
b. RACE
c. RICE
d. PAST

62. Compressed _____ is used as a
power source for instruments such as drills, saws,
and other high-speed tools.
a. Oxygen
b. Argon
c. Nitrogen
d. Nitrous oxide

63. Which of the following compressed medical gases
is used as an anesthetic gas?
a. Oxygen
b. Nitrous oxide
c. Argon
d. Carbon dioxide

64. Chemicals that are transferred from larger containers
to smaller containers must be labeled with the exact
information found on the _____.
a. MSDS sheets
b. Original container
c. OSHA regulation sheets
d. Manufacturer's directions

65. _____ is/are known to contain
benzene, hydrogen cyanide, formaldehyde, blood
fragments, and viruses.
a. Peracetic acid
b. Formaldehyde
c. Smoke plume
d. Filters

66. With regard to toxic chemicals in the operating
room, which of the following statements is true?
a. The cumulative effects can be much greater than
the effects of any single exposure.
b. Many of the chemicals are hazardous, but they
usually produce only short-term effects.
c. Guidelines for handling chemicals are designed
to increase the risk of occupational exposure and
associated injuries.
d. Only the emergency department is required to
maintain MSDS for chemicals.

67. Nonresistant materials include
_____.
a. Metal
b. Water
c. Human body
d. All of the above
e. None of the above

CASE STUDIES

Case Study 1

*Read the following case study and answer the questions based on your knowledge of
fire in the operating room.*

You are scrubbed in and helping with an endoscopic procedure. The surgeon has
disconnected the light cord from the endoscope and placed it on the surgical
drapes.

68. What can you tell the surgeon about patient safety to prevent him from doing this
again?

_____

_____

_____

Case Study 2

Read the following case study and answer the questions based on your knowledge of fire in the operating room.

You are searching the OR suite for something that smells as if it might be hot. You see that a C-arm fluoroscopy machine is plugged into the wall. While you are calling the radiology department to come and check out the machine, it bursts into flame.

69. Using the acronym RACE, describe the actions you will take.

R _____

A _____

C _____

E _____

INTERNET EXERCISES

Internet Exercise 1

Go to the Web site www.osha.gov/SLTC/bloodbornepathogens/standards.html. Study the blood-borne pathogen rule and then answer the following questions.

70. What is involved in the rule? _____

_____

_____

71. What did you learn at this Web site that you did not already know about blood-borne pathogens?

_____

_____

_____

Internet Exercise 2

*Using your favorite search engine, research **HGIB**. Then answer the following questions.*

72. What is HGIB? _____

_____

73. For what is it used? _____

_____

16 Case Planning and Intraoperative Routines

Student's Name _____

KEY TERMS

Write the definition for each term.

1. Assignment board _____

2. Biopsy _____

3. Bleeder _____

4. Blunt dissection _____

5. Case planning _____

6. Case setup _____

7. Count _____

8. Culture _____

9. Frozen section _____

10. Implant _____

11. Sharps _____

12. Time out _____

SHORT ANSWERS

Provide a short answer for each question or statement.

13. What are the five categories of surgical procedures?

    a. _____

    b. _____

    c. _____

    d. _____

    e. _____

14. How will you know what your assignment is and whom your preceptor will be in the operating room on your clinical day?

    _____

137

15. What items are typically found on the surgeon's preference card?

_____

_____

_____

_____

_____

16. What is a "suture book?" _____

_____

_____

_____

17. What items are included in a surgical count?

_____

_____

_____

18. Who is responsible for ensuring that no item is left in a patient?

_____

19. When are surgical counts performed?

- _____

- _____

- _____

- _____

- _____

- _____

20. Items are usually counted in a specific order; what is that order?

a.

b.

c.

d.

21. What is included in a time out?

- _____

- _____

- _____

- _____

- _____

22. How can a needlestick be prevented in the operating room?

a. _____

b. _____

c. _____

23. Identification of specimens is a critical aspect of surgery. Each specimen must be identified with the following information:

(1) _____

(2) _____

(3) _____

(4) _____

(5) _____

(6) _____

Chapter **16** **Case Planning and Intraoperative Routines**

Match each person with the correct job.

24. _____ Unsterile team member

25. _____ Who is responsible for labeling the surgical specimen?

26. _____ Who should adjust the surgical lights as needed during the procedure?

27. _____ Who escorts the patient to the operating room from preop holding?

28. _____ Who opens the sterile supplies onto the sterile field as the room is being opened?

29. _____ Who performs the surgical scrub and gowns and gloves themselves?

30. _____ Who is involved in the time out?

31. _____ Whose job is it to maintain a clean and orderly instrument table and sterile field?

32. _____ Who handles and passes instruments?

33. _____ Who initiates the use of a neutral zone?

34. _____ Who signs the surgical count sheet?

35. _____ Who does the surgical count?

36. _____ Who documents the surgical proceedings?

37. _____ Who looks for a missing sponge?

38. _____ Who is directly responsible for receiving and handling specimens on the surgical field?

a. Scrub
b. Circulator
c. Surgeon
d. *All* team members
e. Scrub and circulator

TRUE/FALSE

Indicate whether the statement is true or false.

39. Each person handling the specimen is part of the chain of custody and liable for errors.

_____ True   _____ False

40. Sterile supplies are opened in sequence from small to large.

_____ True   _____ False

41. After the case is opened, the technologist or scrub nurse performs the surgical scrub.

_____ True   _____ False

42. Before organizing and preparing supplies, the surgical technologist should increase the size of the sterile area by draping the Mayo stand.

_____ True   _____ False

43. During the sterile setup, shifting sterile items from one location to another without purpose increases the chance of contamination and is not productive.

_____ True   _____ False

44. Suture set up is not part of the primary set up.

_____ True   _____ False

45. If instrument trays must be stacked, the lightest trays are placed on the bottom.

_____ True   _____ False

46. Irrigation and soaking solutions usually are distributed after the case is underway or just before the case begins.

_____ True   _____ False

47. If only one medication is on the back table, you do not need to label it.

_____ True   _____ False

48. The surgical count is performed systematically and audibly with the circulator and the scrub person participating equally.

_____ True   _____ False

49. Because e surgical count sheet is a legal document, only the circulator is required to sign it.

_____ True   _____ False

50. Time out is a team event and takes place immediately before surgery is started.

_____ True   _____ False

51. Surgery requires extreme concentration.

_____ True   _____ False

52. Only small surgical sponges are sewn or impregnated with a radiopaque strip.

_____ True   _____ False

53. All instruments are passed in their closed (locked) position unless the surgeon requests otherwise.

_____ True   _____ False

                         Chapter **16** **Case Planning and Intraoperative Routines**

Choose the most correct answer to complete the question or statement.

54. Which of the following specimens might be sent to the pathologist on a Telfa sponge?
    a. Adenoid tissue
    b. Prostate from a TURP
    c. Uterus and fallopian tubes
    d. Breast tissue for frozen section

55. Which of the following specimen must be sent to the pathologist dry?
    a. Colon polyps
    b. Bronchial washings
    c. Kidney stones
    d. Tonsils

56. Excessive or rough handling of bowel tissue can cause a sympathetic nervous response called
    _____.
    a. Paralytic ileus
    b. Small bowel obstruction
    c. Ulcerative colitis
    d. Diverticulitis

57. _____ instruments are passed firmly.
    a. Eye instruments
    b. Orthopedic surgery
    c. Plastic surgery
    d. General surgery

58. Which sponge is used to make a sponge stick?
    a. Laparotomy
    b. 4 × 4
    c. Kittner
    d. Tonsil

59. Which type of sponge is packaged in groups of 10?
    a. Kittner
    b. Cherry
    c. 4 × 4
    d. Laparotomy

60. Which type of sponge would be appropriate for "packing" the abdominal cavity?
    a. Kittner
    b. 4 × 4
    c. Laparotomy
    d. Neuro patties

61. Case planning combines knowledge of
    _____.
    a. Surgical procedure and surgical techniques
    b. Anatomy and pathology
    c. The patient's diagnosis
    d. The patient's prognosis

62. When opening packages sealed with tape, why should you break the tape rather than tear it?
    a. To prevent the outer wrapper from ripping, causing contamination
    b. So that you have to look at the tape to see whether it is sterile
    c. To prevent strike-through
    d. To prevent the inner wrapper from ripping

63. Which of the following is NOT a recommendation for opening a case?
    a. Open the scrub's gown and gloves on a small table or Mayo stand.
    b. Never unwrap a heavy item by holding it in midair.
    c. Do not open small sterile items into the genesis instrument tray.
    d. Open extra sutures, special equipment, and implants so that the surgeon does not have to wait for them during the procedure.

64. After the case has been opened, the surgical technologist's next immediate task is to:
    a. Load the knife blade
    b. Dress the Mayo stand
    c. Perform a surgical hand scrub
    d. Organize the instruments

65. Creating a continuous sterile field _____
    a. Makes the instruments easy for the surgeon to reach
    b. Contaminates the back table
    c. Saves steps and motion
    d. Is against AORN standards

66. After finishing the surgical scrub, which task is done next?
    a. Arrange towels, gowns, and gloves in order of use
    b. Gown and glove self
    c. Organize the knife and the instruments
    d. Put all sponges in one location so you are ready to count

67. The selection of suture material is almost always prescriptive, or _____.
    a. Written on the surgeon's case plan ahead of time
    b. Delayed until the surgeon can prescribe the type she wants
    c. Determined only after the surgeon has taken a look at the surgical wound
    d. Delayed until the surgeon has discussed surgical wound closure with the patient.

68. If the count is incorrect, _____.
    a. A radiograph should be taken immediately.
    b. The surgeon should not be bothered.
    c. The surgeon is notified and the count repeated.
    d. The circulator should call the house supervisor for an incident report.

69. A retained item can cause patient injury from all of the following *except* _____.
    a. X-ray exposure sickness
    b. Infection
    c. Organ perforation
    d. Obstruction

70. Immediately after gowning and gloving, the technologist must complete _____.
    a. Scattering the case
    b. The sterile setup or setting up a case
    c. Preparation of the operating room
    d. The surgical count

71. After you scrub and as you first approach the pile of sterile equipment, do not move anything until:
    a. You have a plan.
    b. You count the instruments.
    c. You load the blade on the knife handle.
    d. You move the drapes and put them in order.

CASE STUDIES

Case Study 1

Read the following case study and answer the questions based on your knowledge of case preparation.

It is 6:30 AM, and you are assigned to OR 6 with your preceptor, who has called and said that she will be late because she has a flat tire. She has asked that you go ahead and get the room ready for the day, "pick the case," and then "scatter the room" (which is to place the sterile but unopened packs onto the furniture where they will be opened soon). She does not want you to "open the case" until she gets there to assist you.

72. How do you get the room "ready" for the day?

    _____

    _____

73. What is involved in "picking the case"?

    _____

    _____

74. What are you going to do to "scatter the room"?

    _____

    _____

75. Why does your preceptor NOT want you to open the case until she is present?

    _____

    _____

Case Study 2

Read the following case study and answer the questions based on your knowledge of case preparation.

Think about putting yourself in the surgical technologist's role. Your surgeon has just come in, and you are about to hand him the towel. What is the sequence of events between that sterile towel and the incision?

1. Towels are distributed, and the team members are gowned and gloved.

2. _____

3. _____

4. _____

5. _____

6. _____

7. The incision is made.

17 The Surgical Wound

Student's Name _____

KEY TERMS

Write the definition for each term.

1. Absorbable suture _____

2. Adhesion _____

3. Anastomosis _____

4. Approximate _____

5. Autotransfusion _____

6. Blunt needle _____

7. Bolster _____

8. Brown and Sharp (B & S) gauge _____

9. Capillary action _____

10. Chromic salt _____

11. Collagen _____

12. Continuous suture _____

13. Contracture _____

14. Debridement _____

15. Dehiscence _____

16. Double-arm suture _____

17. Evisceration _____

18. Fistula _____

19. Inert _____

20. Interrupted suture _____

21. Keloid _____

22. Ligate _____

23. Memory _____

24. Monofilament suture _____

25. Multifilament suture _____

26. Nonabsorbable sutures _____

27. Pliability _____

28. Purse-string suture _____

29. Retention suture _____

30. Reverse cutting needle _____

31. Running suture _____

32. Scar _____

33. Secondary intention _____

34. Swage _____

35. Tensile strength _____

36. Third intention _____

37. Tie on a passer _____

38. Tissue drag _____

SHORT ANSWERS

Provide a short answer for each question or statement.

39. Successful management of the surgical wound is based on five essential principles. What are they?

    (1) _____

    (2) _____

    (3) _____

    (4) _____

    (5) _____

40. What are the guidelines for placement of a surgical tourniquet?

    _____

    _____

    _____

41. What physical injury can be done to the surgical patient if a surgical tourniquet is not used properly?

    _____

42. All substances, including suture products, that bear the USP label must meet minimum standards. What are the

    standards for sutures? _____

    _____

    _____

43. List the five characteristics of sutures that influence a surgeon's decision in choosing a suture.

   a. _____

   b. _____

   c. _____

   d. _____

   e. _____

44. List all the suture materials that have *no* inflammatory properties. _____

_____

45. Describe the types of suture needles. _____

_____

_____

The following is a list of names of alternate and not well known or infrequently used grafting materials. Explain what each is and the purpose for which it is used.

46. Amniotic membrane _____

_____

47. Engineered skin substitutes _____

_____

48. Biobrane _____

_____

49. TransCyte _____

_____

50. Integra Bilayer Matrix Wound Dressing _____

_____

_____

51. Integra Dermal Regeneration Template _____

_____

_____

52. Cultured epithelial autograft _____

_____

_____

53. Foreskin grafts _____

_____

_____

54. What are the purposes of wound dressings?

• _____

• _____

• _____

• _____

• _____

LABELING

Label the following pictures with the type of suture technique shown.

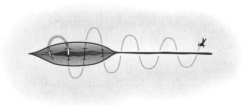

55. _____

57. _____

56. _____

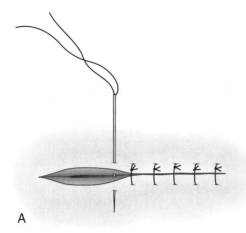

A

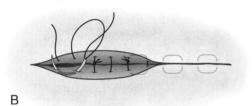

B

58. _____

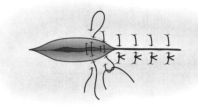

59. _____

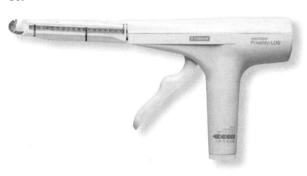

60. _____

Label the following picture of surgical staplers and clip appliers.

61.

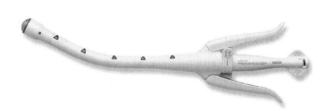

a. _____   b. _____

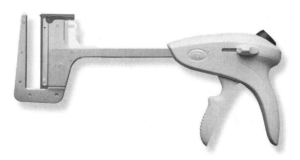

c. _____

Courtesy United States Surgical Corp., Norwark, Conn.

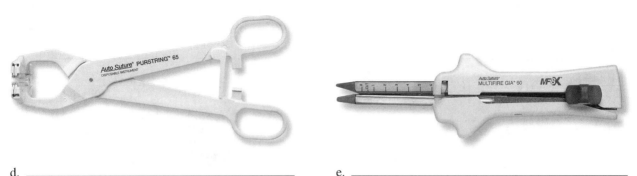

d. _____   e. _____

Courtesy United States Surgical Corp., Norwalk, Conn.

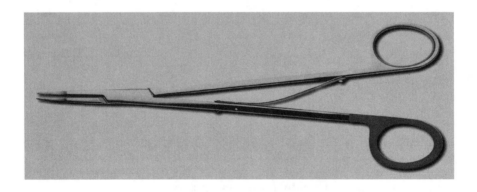

62. _____

Courtesy Week Industries, Research Triangle Park, N.C.

MATCHING I

Match each term with the correct definition as it applies to implants and grafts.

63. _____ Tissue used to cover large defects in the skin
64. _____ Any type of tissue replacement or device placed in the body
65. _____ Tissue graft derived from human tissue
66. _____ Graft taken from pig tissue
67. _____ Tissue obtained from the patient's body and implanted in another site
68. _____ Graft taken from a species different from that of the donor
69. _____ Migration of epithelial cells into the wound during healing
70. _____ Bone graft taken from the hip for implantation in the spine of the same patient

a. Allograft
b. Autograft
c. Bovine graft
d. Epithelialization
e. Implant
f. Porcine graft
g. Xenograft
h. Wound cover

Match each term with the correct definition as it applies to hemostatic drugs and agents.

71. _____ When applied to oozing tissue, this product combines with fibrinogen to promote coagulation.

72. _____ This product is used on bleeding bone.

73. _____ This product may be soaked in normal saline or topical thrombin or used in dry form.

74. _____ The brand name of this product is Surgicel.

75. _____ This powder is applied directly to an oozing surface or mixed with injectable isotonic saline for use as a spray or for soaking hemostatic sponges.

76. _____ This product is never injected into blood vessels.

77. _____ When applied to tissue, this product absorbs blood quickly and forms an artificial clot.

78. _____ This product is available in squares that are cut to size as needed.

79. _____ The unused pieces of this product must be kept away from the surgical wound.

80. _____ The brand name of this product is Avitene.

81. _____ This product is available in mesh.

82. _____ This product must be warmed slightly before use.

a. Thrombin

b. Absorbable gelatin

c. Oxidized cellulose

d. Collagen absorbable hemostat

e. Bone wax

TRUE/FALSE

Indicate whether the statement is true or false.

83. Blood can be a barrier to healing, because it forms a physical barrier between tissue edges.

_____ True   _____ False

84. When significant blood loss is anticipated before surgery, patients may elect to bank their own blood for infusion in the intraoperative or postoperative period.

_____ True   _____ False

85. Autotransfusion and Cell Saver are the same thing.

_____ True   _____ False

86. A pneumatic tourniquet is used to create a bloodless surgical site.

_____ True   _____ False

87. Suture packages are color coded by needle type.

_____ True   _____ False

88. The capillary action of sutures is also sometimes called *wicking*.

_____ True   _____ False

89. With regard to suture size, the greater the diameter, the larger the designated size.

_____ True   _____ False

90. The absorption rate of a surgical suture describes how the suture reacts in the presence of body tissue.

_____ True   _____ False

91. Absorbable, protein-based sutures are attacked by enzyme-releasing lysosomes that digest the suture.

_____ True   _____ False

92. Bioactivity describes the suture's response to the patient's body.

_____ True   _____ False

93. Some multifilament suture is coated to reduce tissue drag and wicking.

_____ True   _____ False

94. Silk suture begins to break down in the patient after about a year and is usually absent from tissue after 2 years.

_____ True   _____ False

95. Surgeons may choose to place a surgical drain, because the presence of fluid in a surgical wound can delay healing and cause infection.

_____ True   _____ False

96. All but very simple drainage systems require a reservoir to collect the fluid.

_____ True   _____ False

97. An example of a closed drainage system is the ½-inch Penrose drain.

_____ True   _____ False

MULTIPLE CHOICE

Choose the most correct answer to complete the question or statement.

98. Conserving the body's total blood volume necessary for life is called _____.
    a. Coagulation
    b. Ligation
    c. Homeostasis
    d. Hemostasis

99. Uncontrolled oozing or insecure hemostasis can lead to a(an) _____.
    a. Hematoma
    b. Contusion
    c. Seroma
    d. Compartment syndrome

100. Which of the following statements is true regarding the formation of a clot?
    a. The blood vessel retracts and constricts.
    b. Even in severe trauma, the body's natural mechanisms control bleeding.
    c. A meshwork of fibrin strands forms around the blood cells.
    d. Once initiated, the clotting cascade takes one route to form a clot.

101. Collection of the patient's blood from the surgical site intraoperatively and intravenous return of the blood is called _____.
    a. Coagulation
    b. Autotransfusion
    c. Hemostasis
    d. Cell Saver

102. Suture materials are used for all of the following *except* _____.
    a. Approximation
    b. Ligation of tubular structures
    c. Hemostasis
    d. Coagulation

103. Which of the following is the *largest* suture type?
    a. #1 Ethibond
    b. #0 silk
    c. 3-0 Vicryl
    d. 11-0 chromic

104. The physical characteristics of suture include which of the following?
    a. Size
    b. Elasticity
    c. Memory
    d. Effect of the suture on the tissue

105. Which of the following suture terms indicates multiple intertwined strands?
    a. Monofilament
    b. Multifilament
    c. Braided
    d. Twisted

106. The _____ of suture refers to the amount of force needed to break the suture.
    a. Knot strength
    b. Tensile strength
    c. Tissue drag
    d. Biological environment

107. Which type of suture is absorbed rapidly in the presence of infection and is not used in contaminated wounds?
    a. Silk
    b. Vicryl
    c. Ethibond
    d. Chromic

108. _____ sutures are no longer marketed in the United States because they have been replaced by more inert materials.
    a. Silk
    b. Cotton
    c. Chromic
    d. Biosyn

109. A wound that is not sutured and must heal from the base is healing by _____.
    a. Delayed union
    b. First intention
    c. Second intention
    d. Third intention

110. Which of the following is the first phase of wound healing?
    a. Healing phase
    b. Remodeling phase
    c. Proliferative phase
    d. Inflammatory phase

111. Which of the following is NOT considered risk factors in wound healing?
    a. Nutritional status
    b. Chronic disease
    c. Obesity
    d. Site of the incision

112. Tissue breakdown at the wound margins is called _____.
    a. Dehiscence
    b. Evisceration
    c. Enucleation
    d. Surgical wound infection

Case Study 1

Read the following case study and answer the question based on your knowledge of surgical tourniquets.

Your surgical patient is going to arrive to the operating room soon for a total knee replacement. You know that the surgeon will require a surgical tourniquet for the procedure. What safeguards are in place to keep your patient safe during the time the tourniquet is being placed and used?

113. _____

114. _____

115. _____

116. _____

117. _____

118. _____

119. _____

120. _____

121. _____

122. _____

123. _____

Case Study 2

Making a suture square: Using the squares below, categorize the sutures from the text. After you have finished that, use a colored pencil to make the suture name in the same color as the suture package.

	Synthetic sutures	Natural sutures
Absorbable sutures		
Nonabsorbable sutures		

Internet Exercise 1

Go online to research a new suture called Tephaflex. The suture is made from patented recombinant DNA technology through the company Tepha, Inc. The company's Web site is: http://www.tepha.com. After researching the site, answer the following questions.

124. How long has the suture been available? _____

125. Does the company make other medical products? _____

126. Is this synthetic suture absorbable or nonabsorbable? _____

127. How does the suture compare to other sutures in the same category as far as tensile strength and other suture

     properties? _____

     _____

128. Is the suture in use today? _____

129. Which type of surgical procedure specialties are being targeted for this type of suture?

     _____

130. Is there a contraindication for use of this suture? _____

     _____

Internet Exercises 2

Using your favorite search engine, research one of the surgical pioneers, William Halstead. Read about his life, his surgical contributions, and his contributions to the way we suture wounds. Why are William Halstead's contributions still significant today? Look for a picture of him. Once you are done researching, write what you learned about this pioneer of surgery that you had not learned from the text.

_____

_____

_____

_____

_____

_____

18 Biomechanics and Computer Technology

Student's Name _____

KEY TERMS

Write the definition for each term as it applies to matter.

1. Atomic number _____

2. Atomic weight _____

3. Boiling point _____

4. State of matter _____

5. Subatomic particles _____

Write the definition for each term as it applies to motion.

6. Momentum _____

7. Electromagnetic field _____

8. Electromagnetic waves _____

Write the definition for each term as it applies to energy.

9. Energy _____

10. Force _____

11. Mechanics _____

12. Potential energy _____

13. Reflection _____

Write the definition for each term as it applies to electricity.

14. Circuit _____

15. Conductivity _____

16. Cycle _____

17. Electric generator _____

18. Electrostatic discharge _____

19. Ground wire _____

20. Hot wire _____

21. Impedance _____

22. Insulator _____

23. Magnetism _____

24. Receptacle _____

25. Resistance _____

157

26. Transformer _____

27. Voltage _____

Write the definition for each term as it applies to light.

28. Focal point _____

29. Photon _____

30. Refraction _____

31. Refractive index _____

32. Serial lenses _____

Write the definition for each term as it applies to sound.

33. Doppler effect _____

34. Doppler ultrasound _____

35. Ultrasound _____

Write the definition for each term as it applies to computer technology.

36. Database _____

37. Flaming _____

38. Hardcopy _____

39. Hard disk drive _____

40. Hyperlink _____

41. LCD _____

42. Menu _____

43. Monitor _____

44. Saving (data) _____

45. Software _____

46. Taskbar _____

47. Toolbar _____

48. Touch screen _____

49. Window _____

50. Word processing _____

SHORT ANSWERS

Provide a short answer for each question or statement.

51. What are the four states of matter? _____.

52. What is the difference between the law of inertia and Newton's law of motion?

_____

_____

_____

53. What is the difference between direct and alternating current? _____

_____

_____

LABELING

54. Label the chart below using the following terms:

    (a) amplitude

    (b) circumference

    (c) crest

    (d) frequency

    (e) peak

    (f) projectile motion

    (g) trough

    (h) waves

    (i) wavelength

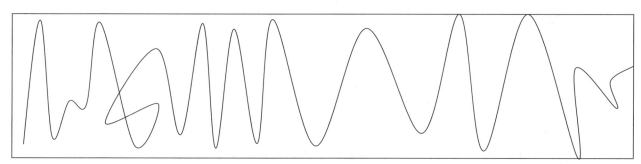

Graph indicates 1 second in time.

MATCHING I

Match each term with the correct definition as it applies to heat.

55. _____ The term for different substances having differing abilities to conduct or transmit heat.

56. _____ Creates a current as the warm air rises and cool air falls

57. _____ The ability of a substance to conduct heat.

58. _____ The transfer of heat by electromagnetic waves.

59. _____ The displacement of cool air by warm air.

60. _____ A complex physiological process in which the body maintains a temperature that is optimal for survival.

61. _____ The transfer of heat from one substance to another by the natural movement of molecules, which sets other molecules in motion.

a. Conduction

b. Convection

c. Radiation

d. Thermal conductivity

e. Thermoregulation

Chapter **18** **Biomechanics and Computer Technology**

Match each term with the correct definition as it applies to matter.

62. _____ A pure substance composed of atoms, each with the same number of protons.

63. _____ A positively charged subatomic particle that is part of the nucleus of an atom.

64. _____ One of the three states or properties of a substance in which the temperature reached the melting point.

65. _____ A state of matter in which the molecules are bonded very tightly.

66. _____ A discrete unit made of matter consisting of charged particles.

67. _____ A charge particle created when an atom loses or gains an electron.

68. _____ An atom of a specific element with the correct number of electrons and protons but a different number of neutrons.

69. _____ A specific substance made up of elements that are bonded together.

70. _____ A subatomic particle located in the nucleus of the atom. The neutron has no electrical charge.

71. _____ A negatively charged particle that orbits the nucleus of an atom.

a. Atom
b. Isotope
c. Molecule
d. Electron
e. Neutron
f. Element
g. Ion
h. Proton
i. Solid
j. Liquid

TRUE/FALSE

Indicate whether the statement is true or false.

72. A concave lens bends light rays toward the center.

_____ True   _____ False

73. The "nonhuman" aspects of surgical technology draw most heavily from the field of mechanics.

_____ True   _____ False

74. The nucleus or center of the atom has two main particles, the neutron and the proton.

_____ True   _____ False

75. Regardless of the number of electrons or neutrons an atom has, the atomic number of the element remains the same.

_____ True   _____ False

76. The periodic table lists all known elements according to their mass and electronic behavior.

_____ True   _____ False

77. Velocity is the speed of a moving object measured as distance over time.

_____ True   _____ False

78. An example of a wave is a disturbance in the flow of the air.

_____ True   _____ False

79. If waves are not exactly the same, but rather vary in size and shape, they are said to be coherent.

_____ True   _____ False

80. Nearly all biomedical devices require electricity as their power source.

_____ True   _____ False

81. Electricity is formed when electrons move from atom to atom.

_____ True   _____ False

MULTIPLE CHOICE

Choose the most correct answer to complete the question or statement.

82. Free electrons flow through conductive material in a continuous path, each electron "pushing" the one ahead of it. This is called (a) _____.
   a. Circuit
   b. Static electricity
   c. Polarity
   d. Alternating current

83. "The natural attractive force of masses in the universe" defines _____.
   a. Gravitational energy
   b. Kinetic energy
   c. Chemical energy
   d. Nuclear energy

84. Which of the following is smallest?
   a. Electron
   b. Proton
   c. Neutron
   d. Atomic nucleus

85. The atomic number of an element corresponds to the element's _____.
   a. Number of electrons
   b. Number of protons
   c. Number of neutrons
   d. Placement on the periodic table

86. Organic compounds all have molecules that contain the element _____.
   a. Iron
   b. Hydrogen
   c. Carbon
   d. Ions

87. "Mass × velocity" is the equation for _____.
   a. Force
   b. Momentum
   c. Distance
   d. Propulsion

88. The distance around a circle is called the _____.
   a. Force
   b. Momentum
   c. Circumference
   d. Projectile motion

89. Potential energy is also referred to as _____.
   a. Energy potential
   b. Electrical energy
   c. Mechanical energy
   d. Stored energy

90. The _____ protects the circuit from a "short" or fault in the system.
  a. Active wire
  b. Neutral wire
  c. Ground wire
  d. Electrical circuit

91. When light rays encounter some surfaces, they can reverse direction; this is called _____.
  a. Refractive index
  b. Refraction
  c. Reflection
  d. Coherence

CASE STUDIES

Case Study 1

Read the following case study and answer the questions based on your knowledge of energy.

Today you are at the park studying for your exam on energy and motion. You notice the children in the park, who are all playing on the toys there. Describe each type of energy or motion exhibited by each of the following children.

Tom and Sally are playing on a teeter-totter.

92. The motion they are exhibiting is _____.

_____.

93. They energy they are exhibiting is _____.

_____.

Jon is playing on a swing set. He is swinging alone.

94. The motion that Jon is exhibiting is _____.

95. The movement is called _____.

Karen and Emily are playing on the merry-go-round.

96. The motion that they are exhibiting is _____.

Jacob is dropping sticks off the bridge into the water.

97. What type of energy is Jacob exhibiting? _____.

Case Study 2

Read the following case study and answer the questions based on your knowledge of computers.

You are going to visit your grandmother today. Grandma has just bought a new computer, and although the computer store technicians came to her house to set it up for her, they did not teach her how to use it, nor did they teach her any of the common terms used in computing. Grandma wants to learn to e-mail her son today. You can help her first by teaching her the following common computer abbreviations.

98. CPU _____

99. RAM _____

100. Disks _____

101. CD _____

102. Cursor _____

103. Icon _____

104. Grandma knows how to type but does not know how to use the mouse. What will you tell her to help her use the mouse?

_____

_____

105. Help Grandma set a password for her computer and show her how to get to the World Wide Web and then to her E-mail provider. Explain the difference between the Internet (which she is not hooked to) and the World Wide Web.

_____

_____

INTERNET EXERCISES _____

Internet Exercise 1

Using your favorite search engine, find a Web site called "How stuff works" and ask, "How does the Internet work?"

106. Describe what you learned.

_____

_____

_____

_____

Give your reference (i.e., the Web site).

_____

Internet Exercise 2

Using your favorite search engine, find a Web site called "How stuff works" and ask, "How does electricity work?"

107. Describe what you watched on the short video.

_____

_____

_____

_____

Give your reference (i.e., the Web site).

_____

Student's Name _____

KEY TERMS

Write the definition for each term.

1. Ablation _____

2. Active electrode _____

3. Active electrode monitoring (AEM) _____

4. Amplification _____

5. Argon _____

6. Bipolar electrosurgery _____

7. Blended mode _____

8. Capacitive coupling _____

9. Capacitive-coupled return electrode _____

10. Carbon dioxide _____

11. Cauterization _____

12. Coagulum _____

13. Coherency _____

14. Conductive _____

15. Continuous wave laser _____

16. Cryosurgery _____

17. Current density _____

18. CUSA _____

19. Cutting mode _____

20. Desiccation _____

21. Direct coupling _____

22. Dispersive electrode _____

23. Electrosurgical unit _____

24. Electrosurgical vessel sealing _____

25. Electrosurgical waveform _____

26. Eschar _____

27. Excitation source _____

28. Excimer _____

29. Fulguration _____

165

30. Grounding pad _____

31. Holmium:YAG _____

32. Implanted electronic device (IED) _____

33. Impedance _____

34. Inactive electrode _____

35. Isolated circuit _____

36. LASER _____

37. Laser classification _____

38. Laser head _____

39. Laser medium _____

40. Lateral heat _____

41. Monochromatic _____

42. Neodymium:YAG _____

43. Optical resonant cavity _____

44. Patient return electrode _____

45. Phacoemulsification _____

46. Potassium-titanyl-phosphate _____

47. Pulsed wave _____

48. Q-switched laser _____

49. Radiant exposure _____

50. Radiofrequency _____

51. Radiofrequency ablation _____

52. Return electrode monitoring _____

53. Selective absorption _____

54. Smoke plume _____

55. Spray coagulation _____

56. Tunable dye _____

57. Ultrasonic energy _____

58. Volt _____

In monopolar electrosurgery, the electrical current passes into the patient's body and makes a complete circuit or a circular path. Label the picture by using the numbers provided.

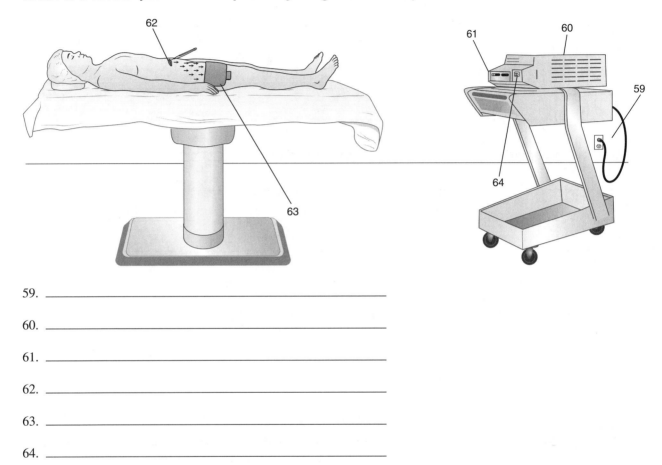

59. _____

60. _____

61. _____

62. _____

63. _____

64. _____

65. In the drawing above, draw in the path of the electrical current. Start with the plug on the wall and draw in a complete circuit.

Provide a short answer for each question or statement.

66. Which variables cause tissue to react to electrosurgery?

    a. _____

    b. _____

    c. _____

    d. _____

67. Describe the difference between cautery, electrosurgery, and ultrasound. _____

    _____

    _____

    _____

    _____

68. What is the difference between monopolar and bipolar delivery of ESU? _____

    _____

    _____

    _____

69. What is captive coupling and why would it occur in endoscopic procedures more often than in open procedures?

    _____

    _____

    _____

    _____

70. How do lasers work? _____

    _____

    _____

    _____

71. How are lasers classified? _____

    _____

    _____

    _____

    _____

72. Lasers are grouped into two categories according to the duration of the output waves. What are the two groups?

a. _____

b. _____

MATCHING I

Match each term with the correct definition.

73. _____ Amount of force that drives electrons through a circuit or pathway.

74. _____ Restriction of electron flow in a direct current circuit.

75. _____ Alternate term for the patient return electrode.

76. _____ Quality of a substance that resists the transfer of electrons and therefore electrical current.

77. _____ In electrosurgery, a continuous path of electricity that flows from the electrosurgery unit to the active electrode, through the patient and return electrode, back to the electrosurgery unit.

78. _____ To cover or surround a conductive substance with nonconductive material.

79. _____ In electricity, the periodicity of electromagnetic waves.

80. _____ In electrosurgery waveforms, the period when the current is actively being delivered.

81. _____ A type of low-voltage current generated by battery.

82. _____ Flow of electricity.

83. _____ Flow of electricity through a conductive medium.

84. _____ Electrical current that changes direction and transmits high-voltage electricity.

a. Current
b. Alternating current
c. Direct current
d. Monopolar circuit
e. Insulate
f. Nonconductive
g. Frequency
h. Neutral electrode
i. Resistance
j. Duty cycle
k. Circuit
l. Voltage

MATCHING II

Match the term with the correct description. Some terms may be used more than once.

85. _____ Invisible to the human eye, and the beam has a high affinity for water.

86. _____ Of all the laser types, has the greatest ability to coagulate blood vessels.

87. _____ A laser that offers two wavelengths, which allows two separate sets of laser characteristics to be selected at any time.

88. _____ This laser beam is outside the visible light range, penetrates all types of tissue, and is extremely versatile.

89. _____ This laser produces a cool beam by stripping electrons from the atoms of the medium in the chamber.

90. _____ This laser beam has a high affinity for tissue protein but little for water.

91. _____ A visible blue-green beam that is absorbed by red-brown pigmented tissue, such as hemoglobin.

92. _____ This pulsed dye laser beam is formed when fluorescent liquid or other dyes are exposed to argon laser light.

a. Argon gas laser
b. Carbon dioxide laser
c. Holmium:YAG laser
d. Nd:YAG laser
e. KTP laser
f. Excimer laser
g. Tunable dye laser

169

Indicate whether the statement is true or false.

93. Because the tissue is burned when an ESU is used, disease transmission through smoke plume is not a risk to surgical personnel.

_____ True   _____ False

94. When working with the ESU, the surgical technologist should not attach the handpiece to the drapes by wrapping it around metal clamps or twisting the cord, because this is a violation of safe use of the ESU.

_____ True   _____ False

95. Argon is inert and nonflammable but easily ionized.

_____ True   _____ False

96. When the ESU tip touches tissue, electricity is impeded, which creates intense heat and produces the desired surgical effect, such as cutting or coagulation.

_____ True   _____ False

97. The return electrode is a pad or thin plate that is placed close to the surgical wound site.

_____ True   _____ False

98. The path of electricity from its origin to destination is the circuit.

_____ True   _____ False

99. The body is very sensitive to high-frequency electricity.

_____ True   _____ False

100. A high-frequency electrocautery current does not interfere with the body's normal functions.

_____ True   _____ False

101. Electrosurgery is the same as cautery.

_____ True   _____ False

102. Monopolar electrocautery is the safest type of electrocautery.

_____ True   _____ False

103. When electricity is applied to the body externally, the tissue reacts according to the voltage and frequency.

_____ True   _____ False

Choose the most correct answer to complete the question or statement.

104. The path of electricity from its origin to destination is the _____
    a. Impedance
    b. Frequency
    c. Circuit
    d. Current

105. Which statement about the body's response to electricity is true?
    a. As the frequency decreases, the body's response increases.
    b. As the frequency decreases, the body's response decreases.
    c. As the frequency increases, the body's response increases.
    d. As the frequency increases, the body's response decreases.

106. _____ electrocautery can cause electrocution or cardiac arrest.
    a. High frequency
    b. Low frequency
    c. Low current
    d. Low voltage

107. _____ is the application of a hot object to living tissue.
    a. Cautery
    b. Electrosurgery
    c. Frequency
    d. Voltage

108. The active electrode is the actual contact point at the tissue and is contained at the:
    a. Tip of the ESU handpiece or "pencil"
    b. Grounding plate
    c. Generator's plug in
    d. Foot pedal

109. The function of the _____ is to capture electrical current from the active electrode and transmit it back to the power unit.
    a. Bipolar
    b. Bayonet
    c. Return electrode
    d. Pencil-type handpiece

110. When the ESU electrode tip touches tissue, electricity is _____, creating intense heat.
    a. Impeded
    b. Volted
    c. Coagulated
    d. Cut

111. Monopolar electrosurgery uses high-voltage _____.
    a. Alternating current (AC)
    b. Direct current (DC)
    c. Voltage
    d. Circuit

112. In the _____ mode, the electrode is held above the tissue, without contact, and the air between the electrode and tissue acts as a conductor, allowing the high-voltage current to flow between the tissue and the electrode.
    a. Blended
    b. Cutting
    c. Desiccation
    d. Microbipolar cutting

113. _____ is therapy in which a probe is inserted into a tumor or tissue mass.
    a. Ultrasound
    b. Phacoemulsification
    c. Cryoablation
    d. Laser

114. When laser light is directed at a surface, which of the following would NOT occur?
    a. Absorption
    b. Coagulation
    c. Reflection
    d. Scattering

Case Study 1

Read the following case study and answer the question based on your knowledge of patient safety when the ESU is used.

Your patient arrives in the preoperative holding area. His history and physical include an implanted electronic device, or IED. Special considerations will be required for his elective surgery, because electrosurgery is planned during the procedure.

What special precautions must be taken to keep this special-population patient safe during his time in the operating room?

115. _____

116. _____

117. _____

118. _____

Case Study 2

Your patient is coming to surgery today, and your surgeon would like to use the laser in her procedure. What safety precautions will the operating room team have to understand and undertake before the laser is used for the patient's procedure?

_____

_____

_____

_____

_____

INTERNET EXERCISES

Internet Exercise 1

Using your favorite search engine, look for the Web site called, "How stuff works." The search is written simply and includes many of your chapter terms and definitions. Once you find the page, ask the following questions in the search box.

119. How do lasers work? (Include chapter terms in your response.)

_____

_____

_____

_____

_____

120. What is a CO_2 laser? (Include chapter terms in your response.)

_____

_____

_____

_____

Internet Exercise 2

Using your favorite search engine, look for the Web site called, "How stuff works." The search is written simply and includes many of your chapter terms and definitions. Once you find the page, ask the following question in the search box.

121. How does electricity work? (Include chapter terms in your response.)

_____

_____

_____

_____

_____

20 Diagnostic and Assessment Procedures

Student's Name _____

KEY TERMS

Write the definition for each term.

1. Acute illness _____

2. Basic metabolic panel _____

3. Benign _____

4. ABO blood groups _____

5. Brachytherapy _____

6. Chemistry test _____

7. Chronic illness _____

8. Complete blood count (CBC) _____

9. Contrast media _____

10. Diastolic pressure _____

11. Differential count _____

12. Doppler studies _____

13. Fluoroscopy _____

14. Electronic probe thermometer _____

15. Endoscopic procedures _____

16. Fibrin _____

17. Frozen section _____

18. Hematocrit (Hct) _____

19. Hemoglobin (Hgb) _____

20. Hypocalcemia _____

21. Hypokalemia _____

22. Hyponatremia _____

23. Imaging studies _____

24. Interstitial needle _____

25. Malignant _____

26. Metastasis _____

27. Neoplasm _____

28. Nuclear medicine _____

29. Orthostatic (postural) blood pressure _____

30. Palpating _____

31. Partial thromboplastin time _____

32. Phase change thermometer _____

33. Prognosis _____

34. Prothrombin time _____

35. Radiopaque_____

36. Radioactive seed _____

37. Radionuclide or isotopes _____

38. Sphygmomanometer _____

39. Sublingual _____

40. Systolic pressure _____

41. TNM classification system _____

42. Transcutaneous _____

43. Tumor marker _____

44. Tympanic membrane thermometer _____

45. Ultrasound energy _____

46. Vital signs _____

SHORT ANSWERS

Provide a short answer for each question or statement.

47. What are the five different ways a patient's temperature might be taken?

    a. _____

    b. _____

    c. _____

    d. _____

    e. _____

48. Explain the three- or four-point scale used to report the strength of the pulse, as well as the terminology used to

describe the pulse. _____

_____

_____

_____

_____

_____

49. Describe the technique for measuring the respiratory rate. _____

_____

_____

50. Describe the technique of evaluating the pulse using the associated terms and definitions and using a three- or

four-point scale. _____

_____

_____

_____

51. What is the technique for measuring the respiratory rate? _____

_____

_____

52. What problems are associated with evaluation of a patient's blood pressure using a simple (digital) automated

sphygmomanometer? _____

_____

_____

_____

53. The CBC is a basic test used to evaluate the type and percentage of normal components in the blood. What five
components are tested?

a. _____

b. _____

c. _____

d. _____

e. _____

54. Positively charged electrolytes are called *cations*. Which cations are routinely tested during a routine blood workup?

_____

55. A routine urinalysis tests specifically for what? _____

_____

_____

Chapter **20**   **Diagnostic and Assessment Procedures**

56. List the different types of pathology tissues. _____

_____

_____

_____

_____

MATCHING I

Match each term with the correct definition.

57. _____ A test that allows physicians to obtain cross-sectional radiographic views of the patient.

58. _____ Medical assessment procedures in which radiographs are used; usually require invasive procedures combined with radiographic technology.

59. _____ A type of medical imaging that measures a specific type of metabolic activity in the target tissue.

60. _____ The average amount of pressure exerted throughout the cardiac cycle.

61. _____ Removal of a sample of tissue for pathologic analysis.

62. _____ A microbiologic study in which cells or fluid are allowed to incubate and then tested for infectivity and sensitivity to an antibacterial agent.

63. _____ A medical device that receives signals from the heart's electrical activity through conductive pads and displays the activity on a graph in real time.

64. _____ A diagnostic technique that uses radiofrequency signals and magnetic energy to produce images.

a. Biopsy

b. C&S

c. ECG

d. EEG

e. MRI

f. PET

g. MAP

h. Interventional radiology

i. CT

MATCHING II

Match each term with the correct definition.

65. _____ Uses radiofrequency signals and multiple magnetic fields to produce a high-definition image.

66. _____ Combines radiography with an image intensifier that is visible in normal lighting.

67. _____ Radiographic and computer technologies are combined to produce high-contrast cross-sectional images.

68. _____ Uses combined technologies to produce an image of a metabolic process in the body rather than a structure.

69. _____ Provides transcutaneous (through the skin) measurement of vascular obstruction.

70. _____ Energy is high-frequency sound waves.

71. _____ Involves the use of radioactive particles, which are directed at the nucleus of a selected element to create energy.

a. MRI

b. Positron emission tomography

c. Doppler

d. Ultrasound

e. Computed tomography

f. Fluoroscopy

g. Nuclear medicine

178

TRUE/FALSE

Indicate whether the statement is true or false.

72. Noninvasive procedures are limited to skin contact or no direct contact with the body.

   _____ True   _____ False

73. Taking the patient's vital signs provides an overall evaluation of well-being.

   _____ True   _____ False

74. The oral temperature is measured sublingually.

   _____ True   _____ False

75. Vital signs remain normothermic regardless of the environmental temperature.

   _____ True   _____ False

76. The stroke volume is the amount of blood pumped through the heart with each heartbeat.

   _____ True   _____ False

77. Blood pressure can be measured in several locations on an arm or a leg.

   _____ True   _____ False

78. The EEG measures the electrical activity of the heart and displays it on a graph for evaluation.

   _____ True   _____ False

79. The term *radiopaque* refers to substances that radiographic rays can easily penetrate, producing a radiograph of the anatomic structure.

   _____ True   _____ False

80. A neoplasm or tumor is a cancerous growth.

   _____ True   _____ False

MULTIPLE CHOICE

Choose the most correct answer to complete the question or statement.

81. _____ is the most basic form of assessment.
   a. CT scan
   b. Chest radiograph
   c. ECG
   d. Vital signs

82. The body requires a core (deep) temperature of approximately 99° F, or _____.
   a. 37.2° C
   b. 38.2° C
   c. 40° C
   d. 42° C

83. Axillary temperature readings are _____ than oral measurements.
    a. 0.3° to 0.6° C higher
    b. 0.5° to 1° F lower
    c. .5° C and 1.5° C lower
    d. 0.6° C and 1.6° C higher

84. _____ varies with environmental changes.
    a. Forehead or skin temperature
    b. Blood pressure
    c. Pulse rate
    d. Pulse oximetry

85. Which statement about the use of thermometers is true?
    a. The use of external thermometers, such as the tympanic thermometer, poses less risk of infection for your patient.
    b. You do not need to wash your hands after taking a patient's temperature with a forehead or skin thermometer because it is not an invasive procedure.
    c. The rectal method is preferred over the tympanic method.
    d. Tympanic thermometers can harbor an infectious biofilm that may not be visible.

86. The pulse is a reflection of the stroke volume, or _____, of each heartbeat.
    a. Amount of input
    b. Amount of oxygen in the blood
    c. Amount of blood pumped through the heart
    d. Amount of blood pumped from the heart into the aorta

87. The normal pulse rate for an adult is _____.
    a. 40 to 60 beats per minute
    b. 60 to 100 beats per minute.
    c. 75 to 110 beats per minute
    d. 80 to 120 beats per minute

88. A bradycardic pulse is described as _____.
    a. 40 to 60 beats per minute
    b. 60 to 100 beats per minute.
    c. 75 to 110 beats per minute
    d. 80 to 120 beats per minute

89. _____ provides detailed information about heart conduction.
    a. ECG
    b. EEG
    c. Blood pressure
    d. Oximetry

90. The basic metabolic panel includes all of the following *except:*
    a. Blood glucose
    b. Carbon dioxide
    c. Creatinine
    d. Oxygen

91. _____ is performed to assess the functional ability of the coagulation sequence.
    a. Electrolyte testing
    b. ABO group testing
    c. PTT
    d. Measurement of ABG levels

CASE STUDIES

Case Study 1

Read the following case study and answer the questions based on your knowledge of temperature conversion.

Your patient is being admitted to the preoperative holding area. The anesthesiologist wants to know the patient's temperature in Celsius, and the temperature is listed on the chart on in Fahrenheit. You will have to do the conversion.

92. What is the conversion from Fahrenheit to Celsius? _____

93. What is the conversion from Celsius to Fahrenheit? _____

94. What do you report back to the anesthesiologist if the patient's temperature is

    written on the chart as 89° F?_____

Case Study 2

Your patient has a cancerous growth. Your task today is to discuss with your patient the specific injury to his body that the malignancy causes. Explain how you would do this; be specific.

_____

_____

_____

_____

INTERNET EXERCISES

Internet Exercise 1

Using your favorite search engine, type in the key words listed below, one at a time, and then answer the questions about each type of pathology exam.

(1) Culture and sensitivity

(2) Tissue biopsy

95. Why is the exam done?

(1) _____

(2) _____

96. Are there specialized instruments, equipment, or solutions used in the exam?

(1) _____

(2) _____

97. How long does the exam take?_____

(1) _____

(2) _____

98. What information did you find about the tissue from the exam?

(1) _____

(2) _____

99. List your Internet sites.

(1) _____

(2) _____

Chapter **20** **Diagnostic and Assessment Procedures**

21 Minimally Invasive Endoscopic and Robotic-Assisted Surgery

Student's Name _____

KEY TERMS

Write the definition for each term.

1. Abdominal adhesions _____

2. Active electrode monitoring (AEM) _____

3. Arthroscopy _____

4. Articulated _____

5. Auxiliary water channel _____

6. Balloon dissector _____

7. Biopsy channel _____

8. Capacitative coupling _____

9. Capacitor _____

10. Control head _____

11. Diagnostic endoscopy _____

12. Direct coupling _____

13. Docking _____

14. Elevator channel _____

15. Endocoupler _____

16. Endoscope _____

17. Eyepiece _____

18. Focus ring _____

19. Gain _____

20. High definition _____

21. Imaging system _____

22. Insertion tube _____

23. Instrument channel _____

24. Intracorporeal _____

25. Intravasation _____

26. Knot pusher _____

27. Laparoscopy _____

28. Master controllers _____

29. Minimally invasive surgery _____

30. Morcellization _____

31. Nephroscopy _____

32. Open surgery _____

33. Optical angle _____

34. Pixel _____

35. Resectoscope _____

36. Robot _____

37. Standard definition _____

38. Stereoscopic viewer _____

39. Surgeon's console _____

40. Telesurgery _____

41. Thoracoscopy _____

42. Video cable _____

43. Video printer _____

SHORT ANSWERS

Provide a short answer for each question or statement.

44. Describe the difference between rigid endoscopy and flexible endoscopy. _____

_____

_____

45. What are the advantages to the patient with MIS? _____

_____

_____

46. What are the limitations associated with MIS? _____

_____

_____

_____

47. What are the special considerations when prepping and draping for MIS procedures?

_____

_____

_____

48. What are the components of the surgical imaging system? _____

_____

_____

49. The guidelines for taking care of the fiberoptic cables include:

 • _____

 • _____

 • _____

 • _____

 • _____

 • _____

 • _____

50. What is the procedure for white balancing? _____

_____

_____

_____

51. Describe the process of insufflation. _____

_____

_____

_____

52. What is the procedure for insertion of a Veress needle? _____

_____

_____

53. During which procedures would continuous irrigation be used? _____

_____

54. What are the guidelines for precleaning optical parts and lenses? _____

_____

_____

MATCHING

Match each term with the correct definition.

55. _____ In minimally invasive surgery, the inflation of the abdominal or thoracic cavity with carbon dioxide gas.

56. _____ Refers to the abdomen when it is distended with carbon dioxide gas.

57. _____ In laparoscopic surgery, a type of cannula that is secured to the abdominal wall with sutures.

58. _____ Meaning "outside the body."

59. _____ A device that controls and emits light for delivery in endoscopic procedures.

60. _____ A sharp, rod-shaped instrument used to puncture the body wall.

61. _____ A surgical technique in which tissue is fragmented to permit removal through an endoscopic cannula.

62. _____ Long, narrow instruments used during endoscopic surgery.

63. _____ A hollow tube

64. _____ A spring-loaded needle used to deliver carbon dioxide gas during insufflation.

65. _____ A commercially prepared suture loop used to secure structures during minimally invasive surgery.

66. _____ The fiberoptic light cable that transmits light from the source to the endoscopic instrument.

67. _____ Refers to the rigid lensed instrument used in minimally invasive surgery.

68. _____ Instrument passed through a natural orifice for assessment or surgery of a hollow organ, duct, or vessel.

a. Veress needle
b. Trocar
c. Telescopic instruments
d. Morcellization
e. Light source
f. Ligation loop
g. Light cable
h. Insufflation
i. Pneumoperitoneum
j. Hasson cannula
k. Extracorporeal
l. Telescope
m. Endoscope
n. Cannula

TRUE/FALSE

Indicate whether the statement is true or false.

69. During pelvic procedures, when the patient is placed in the Trendelenburg position, the patient's lung capacity can cause hypotension from increased pressure on the vena cava.

_____ True   _____ False

70. Procedures of the lungs, bronchi, and upper urinary tract are performed with the patient in the lateral position.

_____ True   _____ False

71. During MIS procedures, a malfunction in any one component affects the others and may significantly reduce patient safety.

_____ True   _____ False

72. To prevent an intraoperative fire, always turn the light source to its highest level before disconnecting it from the telescope or light cable.

_____ True   _____ False

73. The fiberoptic light source transmits light to the camera head or telescope.

_____ True   _____ False

74. Fiberoptic bundles are delicate and easily broken.

_____ True   _____ False

75. During video-assisted surgery, digital signals are captured from the video camera and transmitted to a monitor.

_____ True   _____ False

76. The disposable clip applier delivers single clips before the scrub must reload.

_____ True   _____ False

77. During surgery, instruments should be kept as clean as possible, and only normal saline should be used to clean instruments.

_____ True   _____ False

78. An orderly instrument table protects and preserves instruments.

_____ True   _____ False

79. All instruments must pass through a cleaning and terminal decontamination or sterilization process immediately after use.

_____ True   _____ False

80. Only nonconductive, salt-free fluids are used for continuous irrigation.

_____ True   _____ False

81. The most common use of the flexible endoscope is examination or visual exploration and biopsy.

_____ True   _____ False

82. Flexible endoscopy usually is performed in an outpatient setting.

_____ True   _____ False

Chapter 21 Minimally Invasive Surgery

Choose the most correct answer to complete the question or statement.

83. During laparoscopy, the abdomen is insufflated with _____.
    a. Normal saline
    b. Sodium bicarbonate
    c. Carbon dioxide
    d. Carbon monoxide

84. The positions used for MIS procedures depend on the _____.
    a. Patient's age
    b. Type of anesthetic used
    c. Patient's preference
    d. Target tissue and the patient's physiologic condition

85. The _____ is composed of many thousands of glass or plastic fibers, which are aligned in parallel longitudinal bundles.
    a. Fiberoptic cable
    b. Camera cord
    c. Telescopic lens
    d. Light source

86. Which of the following describes the endocoupler?
    a. Receptacle for the camera
    b. Circuit used in video endoscopy
    c. Connects the camera to the telescope
    d. Clarifies the endoscopic image

87. Your surgeon will need the resectoscope if she is performing a (an) _____.
    a. Orchectomy
    b. Prostatectomy
    c. Laparoscopy
    d. Bilateral oophorectomy

88. Which of the following is considered a rigid telescope?
    a. Laryngoscope
    b. Bronchoscope
    c. Laparoscope
    d. Sigmoidoscope

89. Which of the following endoscopic procedures requires a port for infusing normal saline into the cavity or joint?
    a. Bronchoscopy
    b. Laparoscopy
    c. Arthroscopy
    d. Laryngoscopy

90. Which of the following endoscopic procedures would require infusion of CO_2 into the cavity or joint?
    a. Bronchoscopy
    b. Laparoscopy
    c. Cystoscopy
    d. Arthroscopy

91. An endoscopic instrument, such as a probe or hook, is classified as a _____.
    a. Grasper
    b. Forceps
    c. Scissor
    d. Retractor

92. All rigid endoscopic instruments must pass through _____ immediately after use.
    a. Manual inspection
    b. Cleaning and terminal decontamination process
    c. Sterilization process
    d. Leak test

93. Expansion of the abdominal cavity to expand the body wall and allow clear viewing of the abdominal viscera is called _____.
    a. Infiltration
    b. Insufflation
    c. Continuous irrigation
    d. Balloon expansion

Case Study 1

Read the following case study and answer the question based on your knowledge of telescopes.

You are scrubbed in on a laparoscopic procedure that is about to finish. Your responsibility as a surgical technologist is to properly handle and care for the laparoscope. What does that include?

94. _____

_____

95. _____

_____

96. _____

_____

97. _____

_____

98. _____

_____

Case Study 2

Your surgical patient is undergoing a hysteroscopy. As an educated scrub tech, you know that you must use only nonconductive, salt-free fluids for the continuous irrigation that will be required to perform the procedure.

99. What solutions might your surgeon choose to meet these qualifications?

_____

_____

100. One of the risks involved in these procedures is intravasation. What is intravasation?

_____

_____

101. What injury is involved in intravasation?

_____

_____

102. Who is responsible for keeping track of the fluid inflow and output in these procedures?

_____

_____

INTERNET EXERCISES

Internet Exercise 1

Using your favorite search engine, look for a site called "How stuff works." Type the following questions in the search box and then write what you learn.

103. How does electricity work?

_____

_____

104. What is coupling?

_____

_____

Internet Exercise 2

Using your favorite search engine, research the **Da Vinci Surgical System.** *Then answer the following questions.*

105. At what site did you find the most information about the robotic system?

_____

_____

106. What are the advantages of using robots in surgery?

_____

_____

107. What are the risks of using robots in surgery?

_____

_____

108. What did you find in your research about who developed the first surgical robot?

_____

_____

109. What did you find out about the instruments used in robotic surgery and the classifications of those instruments?

_____

_____

110. What did you find out about the role of the surgical technologist in robotic procedures?

_____

_____

Indicate whether the statement is true or false.

47. Smooth forceps (no teeth) are used on delicate tissue such as serosa, bowel, blood vessels, or ducts.

_____ True   _____ False

48. An example of a bone clamp is the Lane.

_____ True   _____ False

49. If all body tissues were the same, there would be far fewer instruments.

_____ True   _____ False

50. An example of friable tissue is breast tissue.

_____ True   _____ False

51. Familiarity with the body's tissue planes gives the scrub a greater appreciation of the surgical techniques required.

_____ True   _____ False

52. Right-angle scissors, such as Potts scissors, allow the surgeon to insert the scissor tip inside a vessel.

_____ True   _____ False

53. One of the technical goals of surgery is to handle tissue as little as possible.

_____ True   _____ False

MULTIPLE CHOICE: INSTRUMENT IDENTIFICATION

Choose the correct identification or answer to correspond with the picture or question.

54. An example of an angled instrument is a(an) _____.

    a. Schnidt
    b. Right angle
    c. Osteotome
    d. Deaver

55. This instrument penetrates the tissue rather than just holding it.

    a. Tenaculum
    b. Babcock
    c. Kelly
    d. Lowman

56.

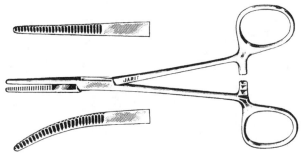

Courtesy Jarit Instruments, Hawthorne, NY.

a. Allis clamp
b. Babcock clamp
c. Kelly hemostat
d. Kocher biting clamp

57.

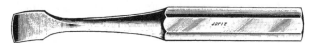

Courtesy Jarit Instruments, Hawthorne, NY.

a. Cushing joker
b. Cup curette
c. Cob elevator
d. Key elevator

58.

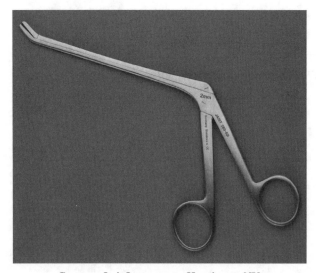

Courtesy Jarit Instruments, Hawthorne, NY.

a. Rongeur
b. Osteotome
c. Curette
d. Shears

59.

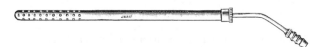

Courtesy Jarit Instruments, Hawthorne, NY.

a. Poole suction tip
b. Yankauer suction tip
c. Frazier suction tip
d. Joseph suction tip

60.

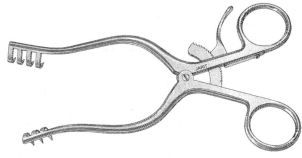

Courtesy Jarit Instruments, Hawthorne, NY.

a. Finochietto
b. Balfour
c. Gelpi
d. Weitlaner

61.

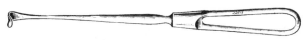

Courtesy Jarit Instruments, Hawthorne, NY.

a. Army-Navy retractor
b. Cushing vein retractor
c. Goelet retractor
d. Richardson retractor

62. What classification is the instrument pictured?

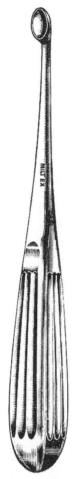

Courtesy Miltex, York, Pa.

a. Retractor
b. Cutting
c. Forceps
d. Miscellaneous

63.

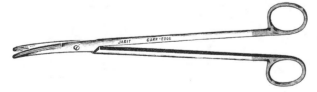

Courtesy Jarit Instruments, Hawthorne, NY.

a. Liston amputation knife
b. Mayo scissors
c. Metzenbaum scissors
d. Babcock clamp

64.

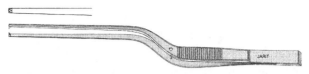

Courtesy Jarit Instruments, Hawthorne, NY.

a. Babcock clamp
b. Bayonet forceps
c. Double-tooth tenaculum
d. Mayo scissors

65.

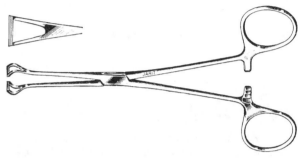

Courtesy Jarit Instruments, Hawthorne, NY.

a. Babcock clamp
b. Duval lung clamp
c. Mosquito hemostat
d. Crile hemostat

Case Study 1

Read the following case study and answer the questions based on your knowledge of surgical instruments.

You are scrubbed in on a vascular case, and your surgeon is about to make an incision into the carotid artery. He will need several instruments in sequence. Using your critical thinking skills, answer the following questions about the instruments.

66. What scalpel blade will your surgeon most likely use to make the incision into the artery?

   _____.

67. What instrument will the surgeon need the very second the incision is made?

   _____.

68. What instrument will the surgeon use to extend the incision?

   _____.

INTERNET EXERCISE

Using your favorite search engine, briefly research the following surgical instruments. Be sure to include the materials of which they are made and the purposes for which they are used.

69. Surgical-grade instruments _____

   _____

   _____

70. Floor-grade instruments _____

   _____

   _____

71. Bright (or mirror) finish instruments _____

   _____

72. Satin finish instruments _____

   _____

73. Ebony finish instruments _____

   _____

74. Disposable instruments _____

_____

_____

75. Resposable instruments_____

_____

_____

23 General Surgery

Student's Name _____

KEY TERMS

Write the definition for each term associated with the abdomen.

1. Abdominal peritoneum _____

2. Direct inguiral repair _____

3. Evisceration _____

4. Fascia (abdominal) _____

5. Fistula _____

6. Hernia _____

7. Hypogastric _____

8. Linea alba _____

9. Mesh _____

10. Paramedian incision _____

11. Pelvic cavity _____

12. Reduce _____

13. Subcutaneous tissue _____

14. Viscera _____

Write the definition for each term associated with the bowel.

15. Anastomosis _____

16. Billroth I procedure _____

17. Bowel technique _____

18. Decompression _____

19. Esophogeal varices _____

20. Exploratory laparotomy _____

21. Gastrostomy _____

22. GERD _____

23. Hiatus _____

24. Laparotomy _____

25. Morbid obesity _____

26. Nasogastric (NG) tube _____

27. Ostomy _____

28. Percutaneous endoscopic gastrostomy tube (PEG) _____
_____

29. Resection _____

30. Stoma _____

31. Stoma appliance _____

Write the definition for each term associated with the liver and spleen.

32. Bifurcation _____

33. Bile _____

34. Biliary system _____

35. Cirrhosis _____

36. Common bile duct exploration (CBDE) _____
_____

37. Friable _____

38. Lobectomy (liver) _____

39. Segmental resection _____

40. Skeletonize _____

41. Subphrenic area _____

42. Transect _____

43. Trisegmentectomy _____

44. Tumor margins _____

Write the definition for each term associated with the breast.

45. Body image _____

46. Frozen section _____

47. Hook wire _____

48. Mastectomy _____

49. Modified radical mastectomy _____

50. Skin flap _____

51. Staging _____

52. Technetium-99 _____

Labeling the Breast

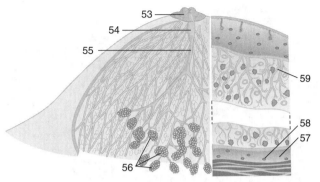

Modified from Donegan WL, Spratt JS: *Cancer of the breast*, Philadelphia, 1988, WB Saunders.

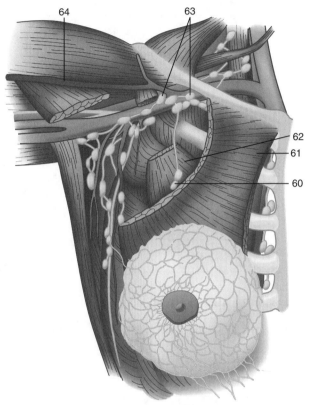

Modified from Donegan WL, Spratt JS: *Cancer of the breast,* Philadelphia, 1988, WB Saunders.

53. _____

54. _____

55. _____

56. _____

57. _____

58. _____

59. _____

60. _____

61. _____

62. _____

63. _____

64. _____

Labeling the Liver

65. _____

66. _____

67. _____

68. _____

69. _____

70. _____

71. _____

72. _____

73. _____

74. _____

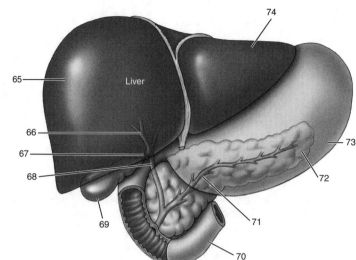

Modified from Herliny B, Maebius NK: *The human body in health and illness*, ed 2, Philadelphia, 2003, WB Saunders.

Labeling for Abdominal Incisions

Draw in the following types of abdominal incisions.

75. Subcostal

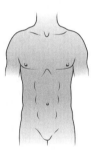

Modified from Rothrock JC: *Alexander's care of the patient in surgery*, ed 12, St Louis, 2003, Mosby.

76. Paramedian

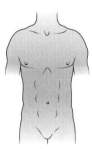

Modified from Rothrock JC: *Alexander's care of the patient in surgery*, ed 12, St Louis, 2003, Mosby.

77. McBurney

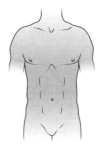

78. Pfannenstiel

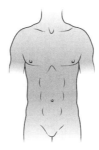

79. Upper midline

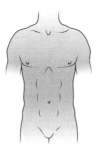

80. Upper abdominal transverse

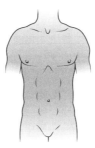

81. Oblique

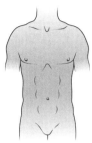

82. Lower midline

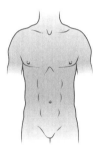

83. Draw the four quadrants of the abdomen and label them.

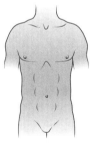

SHORT ANSWER

Provide a short answer for each question or statement.

84. What is the difference between mobilizing tissue and surgically undermining tissue?

_____

_____

85. What are the components of Hesselbach's triangle?

a. _____

b. _____

c. _____

86. What is the difference between a Billroth I and a Billroth II in terms of resection and anastomosis?

_____

_____

_____

_____

MATCHING I

Match each term with the correct definition.

87. _____ Hernia that results from an acquired weakness in the inguinal floor.

88. _____ Herniated tissue that is trapped in an abdominal wall defect.

89. _____ Hernia found in the region of the abdomen above the umbilicus.

90. _____ Abdominal region literally "below the stomach."

91. _____ Postoperative herniation of tissue into the tissue layers an abdominal incision.

92. _____ Hernia that protrudes into the membranous sac of the spermatic cord.

93. _____ Hernia in which abdominal tissue has become trapped between the layers of an abdominal wall defect.

94. _____ Same as an incisional hernia.

a. Ventral hernia

b. Direct inguinal hernia

c. Incisional hernia

d. Incarcerated hernia

e. Hypogastric

f. Epigastric

g. Indirect inguinal hernia

h. Strangulated hernia

MATCHING II

Match each type of breast procedure with the correct definition.

95. _____ Removal of a tissue mass for pathological examination.

96. _____ Also called a simple mastectomy; procedure that removes the breast, including skin, nipple, and lymph nodes.

97. _____ Same as a lumpectomy.

98. _____ Procedure in which tissue surrounding a hook wire device is removed.

99. _____ Procedure that removes the breast while leaving the skin, nipple, and areola intact.

100. _____ Procedure in which one or more lymph nodes are removed to determine whether a tumor has metastasized.

101. _____ The wide breast mass.

102. _____ Procedure that removes breast tissue, including the skin, areola, and nipple.

103. _____ Removal of the entire breast, the nipple, and areola region.

a. Needle localization biopsy

b. Excisional biopsy

c. Lumpectomy

d. Total mastectomy

e. Modified radical mastectomy

f. Sentinel lymph node biopsy

g. Simple mastectomy

h. Subcutaneous mastectomy

i. Segmental mastectomy

Indicate whether the statement is true or false.

104. The body is divided into semiclosed compartments or cavities that contain specific anatomical structures and organs.

_____ True   _____ False

105. Hesselbach's triangle is associated with epigastric hernias.

_____ True   _____ False

106. The McBurney incision is a short, right transverse incision used for appendectomy.

_____ True   _____ False

107. Surgery of the abdominal wall is performed to repair an acquired or congenital defect.

_____ True   _____ False

108. An indirect inguinal hernia arises from the internal inguinal ring and protrudes into the spermatic cord and into the scrotum.

_____ True   _____ False

109. Biosynthetic mesh is made of synthetic material similar to suture, such as Vicryl or Dexon.

_____ True   _____ False

110. An incarcerated hernia is one in which the spermatic cord is trapped between tissue layers.

_____ True   _____ False

111. A femoral hernia results from a weakness in the transversalis fascia.

_____ True   _____ False

112. A ventral hernia is another name for an incisional hernia.

_____ True   _____ False

113. "Bowel technique" is also known as "isolation technique."

_____ True   _____ False

114. The abdomen is divided into four major sections, or landmarks, called *quadrants*.

_____ True   _____ False

115. An ostomy is a procedure in which a portion of the intestine is divided and the open end is secured to the skin, allowing the bowel contents to drain outside the body.

_____ True   _____ False

MULTIPLE CHOICE

Choose the most correct answer to complete the question or statement.

116. Which of the following describes a trisegmentectomy?
    a. A procedure to determine whether stones or a stricture is present in the common bile duct
    b. Removal of one or more anatomical sections
    c. Removal of the right lobe of the liver and a portion of the left
    d. Removal of a small, pie-shaped portion of the liver for biopsy

117. A radioactive substance that is used to identify sentinel lymph nodes is _____.
    a. Technetium
    b. Bile
    c. Cirrhosis
    d. Hiatus

118. Esophageal varices typically are caused by what disease process?
    a. Herniation
    b. Cancer
    c. Cirrhosis
    d. Advanced liver disease

119. Diagnostic endoscopy of the esophagus, stomach, and proximal duodenum is called _____.
    a. Esophagoduodenoscopy
    b. Cholangiogram
    c. Sigmoidoscopy
    d. Gastroscopy

120. Which of the following statements about laparotomy is true?
    a. All loose sponges must be removed from the surgical field.
    b. Only 4 × 4s mounted on sponge forceps are used while the abdomen is open.
    c. Only loose Kittners may be used in the abdomen.
    d. Sponges are not used intra-abdominally.

121. Which of the following statements about endoscopy are true? (Select all that apply.)
    a. The scrub assists the surgeon by guiding the long instruments into the endoscope and handling them when they are withdrawn.
    b. Colonoscopy is endoscopy of the large intestine and is referred to as "upper GI" endoscopy.
    c. Laparoscopy is a surgical procedure in which the abdomen is surgically opened.
    d. Billroth I is a common endoscopic procedure.

122. Resection of the small intestine is performed to treat all of the following *except:*
    a. Obstruction
    b. Ulcer
    c. Inflammation
    d. Carcinoma

123. Which of the following statements regarding APR is true?
    a. In abdominoperineal resection, the anus and rectum are removed one at a time through an abdominal incision.
    b. Two teams may operate simultaneously.
    c. In abdominoperineal resection, the sigmoid colon is removed through the perineal incision.
    d. The anus, rectum, and sigmoid colon are removed en bloc through combined abdominal and perineal incisions.

124. Hemorrhoids occur when _____.
    a. The venous plexus of the anal canal becomes congested or distended.
    b. The anus prolapses outside the anal canal.
    c. The anus begins to bleed.
    d. The arteries of the anus become swollen and engorged with blood.

125. Patients who have esophageal varices _____.
    a. Have end-stage alcoholic liver disease
    b. Have fibrosis of the liver
    c. that rupture in the esophageal venous plexus
    d. All of the above

126. Diseases of the biliary system include all of the following *except:*
    a. Cholelithiasis
    b. Cholecystitis
    c. High blood cholesterol
    d. Obesity

Case Study

You are scrubbed in on an emergency endoscopic appendectomy.

127. What are the exact eight steps (in order) for performing an appendectomy?

(1) _____

(2) _____

(3) _____

(4) _____

(5) _____

(6) _____

(7) _____

(8) _____

INTERNET EXERCISES

Internet Exercise 1

Obesity is an endemic health problem in the United States. It contributes to cardiovascular disease, cancers of the breast and large intestine, diabetes, stroke, urinary stress incontinence, and depression. Approximately 400,000 people die each year in the United States as a result of obesity. Using your favorite search engine, research the effects of obesity in the United States.

128. List your references. _____

_____

_____

129. What did you find? _____

_____

_____

_____

Internet Exercise 2

Occasionally in surgery, the surgical technologist will be asked to dress the wound. If the surgeon has just completed a bowel resection with creation of a colostomy stoma, the dressings will include the placement of the colostomy bag over the newly created stoma. Go online to the International Ostomy Association of America and read the Web page. Then answer the following questions?

130. What is the procedure for dressing the stoma? _____

_____

_____

131. Should the wound or the stoma be dressed first? _____

    Why? _____

    _____

132. Is the colostomy bag sterile? _____

133. If you are using the colostomy paste, is the paste flammable?

    _____

134. If you find that the paste is flammable, what are the guidelines for using the ESU after the paste has been

    applied? _____

    _____

24 Gynecological and Obstetrical Surgery

Student's Name _____

KEY TERMS

Write the definition for each term.

1. Ablate _____

2. Adnexa _____

3. Bladder flap _____

4. Coitus _____

5. Colposcopy _____

6. Cystocele _____

7. Electrolytic media _____

8. En bloc _____

9. Episiotomy _____

10. Fibroid _____

11. Extravasation _____

12. Hysteroscopy _____

13. Incompetent cervix _____

14. Incomplete abortion _____

15. LEEP _____

16. Menarche _____

17. Missed abortion _____

18. Nuchal cord _____

19. Obturator _____

20. Oophorectomy _____

21. Papanicolaou (PAP) test _____

22. Parturition _____

23. Patency _____

24. Perineum _____

25. PID _____

26. Placenta abortion _____

27. Rectocele _____

28. Transcervical _____

29. Uterus _____

Chapter **24 Gynecological and Obstetrical Surgery**

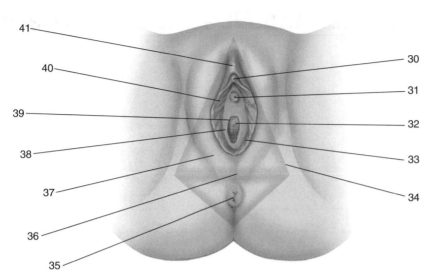

From Thibodeau G, Patton K: *Anatomy and physiology,* ed 6, St Louis, 2007, Mosby.

30. _____   36. _____

31. _____   37. _____

32. _____   38. _____

33. _____   39. _____

34. _____   40. _____

35. _____   41. _____

MATCHING

Match each term with the correct definition.

42. _____ Herniation of the bladder into the vaginal wall.

43. _____ Mass that arises from the germ layers of the embryo that contains tissue remnants, including hair and teeth.

44. _____ Endometrial tissue growth outside of the uterine cavity.

45. _____ Fibrous, benign tumor of the uterus that usually arises from the myometrium.

46. _____ Excessive proliferation of tissue.

47. _____ Sexually transmitted disease or other disease arising from an infection that causes scarring of the fallopian tubes and adhesions in the abdominal and pelvic cavity.

48. _____ Bulging of intestinal tissue into a weakened posterior vaginal wall.

49. _____ Excessive menstrual bleeding.

50. _____ Persistent or bleeding ovarian follicle that fails to regress after ovulation.

51. _____ Diagnosed in women with persistent multiple cystic follicles.

52. _____ Weakness and stretching of the cardinal ligaments that results in uterine prolapse.

53. _____ Implantation of the embryo outside the intrauterine cavity.

a. Ovarian cyst

b. Hyperplasia

c. Polycystic disease syndrome

d. Ectopic pregnancy

e. Uterine prolapse

f. Cystocele

g. Endometriosis

h. PID

i. Rectocele

j. Dermoid cyst

k. Leiomyoma

l. Menorrhagia

Indicate whether the statement is true or false.

54. The Papanicolaou test is performed to screen for cervical cancer.

_____ True _____ False

55. Antiembolism stockings or a sequential pressure device must be worn by all OB/GYN patients.

_____ True _____ False

56. During abdominal procedures, a right-handed surgeon stands at the patient's left side.

_____ True _____ False

57. A complete menstrual cycle is called the *ovarian cycle*.

_____ True _____ False

58. The menstrual cycle is controlled by a complex feedback system involving hormones of the pituitary, hypothalamus, and ovaries.

_____ True _____ False

59. Endometriosis is a condition in which endometrial tissue overdevelops in the uterus.

_____ True _____ False

60. Leiomyoma is a cancerous neoplasm of uterine muscle.

_____ True _____ False

61. Cone biopsy is removal of a circumferential core of tissue around the cervical canal.

_____ True _____ False

62. Endometrial ablation is the destruction of the myometrium.

_____ True _____ False

63. In dilation and curettage (D & C), the surface of the myometrium is removed with sharp and smooth curettes.

_____ True _____ False

64. Placental abruption is the premature separation of the placenta from the uterine wall after 20 weeks of gestation.

_____ True _____ False

Choose the most correct answer to complete the question or statement.

65. Which of the following statements is true regarding lowering a patient's legs from stirrups?
    a. Placing the patient in the lithotomy position may cause changes in the heart rate.
    b. The legs are raised and lowered one at a time only after the anesthesia care provider has advised that it is safe to do so.
    c. Three people are required to move the patient from the stretcher to the OR table.
    d. The move must be performed slowly to prevent injury.

66. Gynecological procedures are performed in the _____ position.
    a. Lateral
    b. Supine
    c. Prone
    d. Kraske

67. _____ is removal of the uterus by a combined laparoscopic and vaginal approach.
    a. PAP
    b. PDS
    c. LAVH
    d. PID

68. _____ involves complete removal of the rectum, the distal sigmoid colon, the urinary bladder and distal ureters, and the internal iliac vessels and their lateral branches.
    a. Radical hysterectomy
    b. Total abdominal hysterectomy
    c. Pelvic exenteration
    d. Partial vaginal hysterectomy

69. _____ is the absorption of hypotonic fluid through the open vessels of the uterus during hysteroscopy.
    a. Extravasation
    b. Hysteroscopy
    c. Cardiac overload
    d. Cardiac output

70. _____ is the removal of a benign tumor.
    a. Vulvectomy
    b. Myomectomy
    c. Hysterectomy
    d. Oophorectomy

71. _____ is the premature separation of the placenta from the uterine wall after 20 weeks of gestation and before the fetus is delivered.
    a. Placenta acreda
    b. Placenta previa
    c. Placental abruption
    d. Umbilical cord prolapse

72. An umbilical cord wrapped one or more times around the baby's neck is called a _____.
    a. Nuchal cord
    b. Prolapsed cord
    c. Premature cord
    d. Cord rope

73. Which of the following is NOT an indication for a C-section for delivery?
    a. Placenta previa
    b. Mother with active herpes outbreak
    c. Prolapsed cord
    d. Labor that lasts longer than 10 hours

74. Ectopic pregnancy occurs when implantation of the fertilized egg:
    a. Occurs outside the uterus
    b. Occurs 8 days after ovulation
    c. Occurs by in vitro fertilization
    d. Fails to occur

75. Risk factors for an ectopic pregnancy include _____.
    a. Previous history of pelvic inflammatory disease (PID)
    b. Smoking (reduces tubal motility)
    c. Previous tubal surgery
    d. All of the above

Case Study 1

Read the following case study and answer the questions.

A complete review of systems (ROS) in your OB/GYN patient includes the following eight components. What exactly does each section include?

76. Menstrual history

    _____

    _____

77. Obstetrical history

    _____

    _____

78. Use of contraceptives

    _____

    _____

79. History of previous infection

    _____

    _____

80. Signs and symptoms

    _____

    _____

81. Current medications and allergies

    _____

    _____

82. Family history

    _____

    _____

83. Social history

    _____

    _____

Gynecology procedures are performed with the patient in the supine or lithotomy position. What are the critical safety considerations for the lithotomy position?

84. _____

85. _____

86. _____

87. _____

88. _____

89. _____

90. _____

INTERNET EXERCISES

Internet Exercise 1

Using your favorite search engine, research abnormal Pap smear results and then answer the following questions.

91. What Web site did you use? _____

_____

92. What are the possible noncancerous abnormal cell results? _____

_____

_____

93. What abnormal cancerous cells are possible? _____

_____

_____

94. What advice did the Web site offer about follow-up physician's visits if abnormal cells are found? _____

_____

_____

25 Genitourinary Surgery

Student's Name _____

KEY TERMS

Write the definition for each term.

1. Arteriovenous fistula or shunt _____

2. Balanitis _____

3. Benign prostatic hypertrophy (BPH) _____

4. Calculi _____

5. Circumcision _____

6. Cystoscope _____

7. Cystoscopy assistant _____

8. Enucleation _____

9. Epispadias _____

10. Extracorporeal shockwave lithotripsy (ESWL) _____

    _____

11. Extravasation _____

12. Foley catheter _____

13. Hematuria _____

14. Hypospadias _____

15. Hypothermia _____

16. Hydronephrosis _____

17. Indwelling catheter _____

18. KUB _____

19. Lithotripsy _____

20. Micturition _____

21. Meatotomy _____

22. Nonelectrolytic _____

23. Percutaneous _____

24. Pyeloplasty _____

25. Resectoscope _____

26. Reflux _____

27. Retrograde pyelography _____

28. Staghorn stone _____

29. Stent _____

30. Straight catheter _____

31. Suprapubic catheter _____

32. Tamponade _____

33. Torsion _____

34. Transurethral_____

35. Urethrotomy _____

SHORT ANSWERS

Provide a short answer for each question or statement.

36. What causes end-stage renal disease (ESRD)? _____

_____

_____

37. UTI is infection of the lower urinary tract and is commonly caused by *Escherichia coli* contamination of the distal

urethra. How does that occur? _____

_____

_____

38. What is dialysis and how does it work? _____

_____

_____

LABELING

Identify the urinary catheters in the following figure, starting left to right.

39. (a) _____

40. (b) _____

41. (c) _____

42. (d) _____

43. (e) _____

44. (f) _____

45. (g) _____

46. (h) _____

47. (i) _____

Modified from Walsh PC, Retik AB, Vaughan Ed et al: *Campbell's urology,* ed 8, Philadelphia, 2002, WB Saunders.

MATCHING

Match each term with the correct definition.

48. _____ A small incision made in the urethra to reduce scaring or relieve a stricture

49. _____ Imaging studies of the renal pelvis that use a contrast medium instilled through a transurethral catheter

50. _____ Reconstruction of the ureter in the renal pelvis

51. _____ A small incision made in the urethral meatus to relieve a stricture

52. _____ Urination

53. _____ A procedure in which ultrasonic sound waves are used to pulverize kidney or gallbladder stones

54. _____ The removal of tissue or an organ without prior fragmentation or dissection

55. _____ Removal of all or part of the prepuce (foreskin) of the penis

56. _____ Inflammation of the glans penis

57. _____ Surgical creation of vascular access for patients undergoing hemodialysis

a. Pyeloplasty
b. Meatotomy
c. Retrograde pyelography
d. ESWL
e. Balanitis
f. Micturition
g. Enucleation
h. Urethrotomy
i. A-V shunt
j. Circumcision

TRUE/FALSE

Indicate whether the statement is true or false.

58. Chronic UTI may result in scarring of the urethra, requiring surgery.

_____ True   _____ False

59. End-stage renal disease (ESRD) is renal failure that cannot be reversed.

_____ True   _____ False

60. Polycystic disease is hereditary, and no treatment is available for it.

_____ True   _____ False

61. Benign prostatic hyperplasia (BPH) is enlargement of the prostate gland related to a disease process.

_____ True   _____ False

62. Hypospadias is a common congenital defect in which the urethra fails to develop fully.

_____ True   _____ False

63. Testicular torsion is a medical emergency.

_____ True   _____ False

64. Varicocele is enlarged dilated veins in the scrotum related to age.

_____ True   _____ False

65. Laboratory tests in genitourinary disease focus on the presence or absence of substances found in the kidneys.

_____ True   _____ False

66. Blood tests such as serum creatinine measure the rate of creatinine in the urine.

_____ True   _____ False

67. The ureters are extremely delicate tissue.

_____ True   _____ False

MULTIPLE CHOICE

Choose the most correct answer to complete the question or statement.

68. Kidney stones are formed by _____ precipitated from filtrate produced in the kidney. Stones are removed to prevent infection and obstruction.
    a. Urine
    b. Crystalline mineral and salts
    c. Lyzed blood cells
    d. Refined bile

69. A UTI is an infection of the lower urinary tract and is commonly caused by _____.
    a. *Streptococcus*
    b. *Pseudomonas*
    c. *E. coli*
    d. *S. aureus*

70. A common genital defect in which the urethra fails to develop fully, resulting in displacement of the urethral meatus on the back side of the penis, is called _____.
    a. Hydronephrosis
    b. Hypospadias
    c. Torsion
    d. Epispadias

71. Varicocele is enlarged dilated veins in the scrotum related to _____.
    a. Venous valve failure
    b. Age
    c. Disease
    d. ESRD

72. During peritoneal dialysis:
    a. The peritoneum acts as a filter to remove metabolic wastes.
    b. The blood is shunted into the heparinized hemodialysis machine.
    c. The blood passes through a series of membranes and dialyzing solution, which filter waste and return the waste to the body.
    d. The solution is returned to the patient's body with the blood.

73. If the surgeon is about to investigate a ureter, which surgical instrument would you hand her?
    a. Kocher
    b. Ferris Smith pickup
    c. Babcock
    d. Carmalt

74. The rigid cystoscope initially is passed through the _____ to perform diagnostic or operative procedures.
    a. Ureter
    b. Bladder neck
    c. Kidney pelvis
    d. Urethral meatus

75. Renal cysts originate in the nephron as a result of _____.
    a. Obstruction
    b. Uremic buildup
    c. Stones
    d. Fluid

76. Which of the following is a medical emergency, because blood flow to the testicle may be obstructed, leading to ischemia and necrosis of the testicle?
    a. Varicocele
    b. Dialysis
    c. Torsion of the testicle
    d. Hypospadias

77. Which of the following urinary system diseases are characterized by the backward movement of urine caused by an obstruction such as a stricture, stone, or tumor?
    a. ESRD
    b. Hydronephrosis
    c. Diabetes
    d. Polycystic disease

78. Imaging tests are performed for all of the following reasons *except* _____.
    a. Outline the structures of the GU system
    b. Observe the function of the GU system
    c. Detect a tumor
    d. Measure the creatinine level

79. The causes of end-stage renal disease include all of the following *except* _____.
    a. Diabetes
    b. Hypertension
    c. Systemic lupus erythematosus
    d. Cysts

CASE STUDIES

Case Study 1

Read the following case study and answer the question based on your knowledge of cystoscopy.

You are about to scrub for a cystoscopy when the OR supervisor delivers a surgical technology student to you and asks you to serve as her preceptor for the case. Your student has never seen a cystoscopy before, and you decide to describe the procedure to her before you start.

80. What steps would you describe to her to explain the procedure?

    (1) _____

    (2) _____

    (3) _____

    (4) _____

    (5) _____

    (6) _____

    (7) _____

    (8) _____

Case Study 2

Read the following case study and answer the question based on your knowledge of irrigation solutions used in GU procedures.

During cystoscopic procedures, the bladder is distended with fluid to enhance visualization of the internal structures. Describe the following solutions, which are commonly used in cystoscopic procedures, and explain when they might be used.

81. Sorbitol _____

82. Glycine _____

83. Sterile distilled water _____

_____

84. Water _____

INTERNET EXERCISES

Internet Exercise 1

Using your favorite search engine, go online and search for innovations underway or being researched concerning GU procedures and biotechnology or stem cells.

_____

_____

_____

_____

_____

_____

_____

26 Ophthalmic Surgery

Student's Name _____

KEY TERMS

Write the definition for each term.

1. Accommodation _____

2. Bridle suture _____

3. Cataract _____

4. Conformer _____

5. Focal point _____

6. Cryotherapy _____

7. Diathermy _____

8. Glaucoma _____

9. Keratoplasty _____

10. Pterygium _____

11. Refraction _____

12. Spatula needle _____

LABELING

Label the following anatomical pictures.

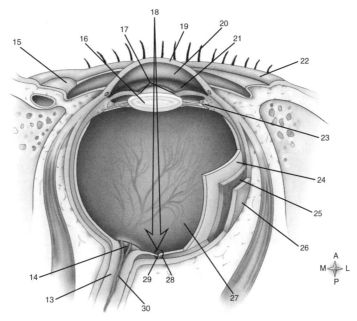

Modified from Thibodeau G, Patton K: *Anatomy and physiology,* ed 6, St Louis, 2007, Mosby.

13. _____ 22. _____

14. _____ 23. _____

15. _____ 24. _____

16. _____ 25. _____

17. _____ 26. _____

18. _____ 27. _____

19. _____ 28. _____

20. _____ 29. _____

21. _____ 30. _____

SHORT ANSWER

Provide a short answer for the question.

31. Lens implants are treated in much the same way as a drug distributed to the field. What does this mean?

_____

_____

_____

_____

MATCHING

Match each term with the correct definition.

32. _____ Surgical removal of a portion of the trabecula to improve outflow of aqueous in the treatment of glaucoma

33. _____ A process in which high-frequency sound waves are used to emulsify tissue, such as a cataract

34. _____ Surgery in which the eye muscle is moved back to release the globe

35. _____ Surgical shortening of an eye muscle to pull the globe into correct position

36. _____ Surgical removal of the globe and accessory attachments

37. _____ Surgical removal of the contents of the eyeball, with the sclera left intact

38. _____ Removal of the entire contents of the orbit

39. _____ A technique in which a cold probe is used to freeze tissue, such as the sclera, ciliary body (for glaucoma), or retinal layers, after detachment

40. _____ Low-power cautery used to mark the sclera over the area of retinal detachment

a. R&R

b. Trabeculectomy

c. Exenteration

d. Diathermy

e. Cryothermy

f. Enucleation

g. Phacoemulsification

h. Muscle recession

i. Evisceration

j. Muscle resection

Indicate whether the statement is true or false.

41. Refraction is a test for visual acuity that is performed with a photo-opter.

    _____ True   _____ False

42. Conray is used to stain the cornea and highlight irregularities of the epithelial surface.

    _____ True   _____ False

43. Fluorescein angiography is used extensively in the diagnosis and evaluation of retinal and choroid disease.

    _____ True   _____ False

44. Skin prep of the eye may include instillation of drugs to prepare the eye for surgery.

    _____ True   _____ False

45. Nearly all eye surgery is performed using a regional anesthetic with monitored sedation.

    _____ True   _____ False

46. A chalazion is a benign inflammatory growth.

    _____ True   _____ False

47. Entropion is drooping of the lower eyelid.

    _____ True   _____ False

48. Dacryocystorhinostomy is the creation of a permanent opening in the tear duct for the drainage of tears.

    _____ True   _____ False

49. It is imperative that the operating room remain stress free during ophthalmic procedures because anxiety can result in increased hemorrhage.

    _____ True   _____ False

50. Creating a reassuring environment is important to the patient's psychological and physical well-being.

    _____ True   _____ False

Choose the most correct answer to complete the question or statement.

51. The slit lamp is used to examine the _____.
    a. Posterior chamber of the eye
    b. Anterior chamber of the eye
    c. Retina
    d. Crystalline lens

52. _____ is used to stain the cornea and highlight irregularities of the epithelial surface.
    a. Fluorescein
    b. Conray
    c. Hypaque
    d. Methylene blue

53. Direct examination of the eyes is performed with the _____.
    a. Surgeon's loupes
    b. Operative microscope
    c. Ophthalmoscope
    d. Bifocals

54. _____ is a test used to measure the density of tissues and detect abnormalities.
    a. Direct examination
    b. Ophthalmic ultrasonography
    c. Fluorescein angiography
    d. Slit lamp examination

55. Muscle resection and recession (R&R) is performed to correct deviation of the eye caused by:
    a. Strabismus
    b. Pterygium
    c. Chalazion
    d. Entropion

56. The surgical goal of scleral buckling is to _____.
    a. Restore the vascular layer of the retina
    b. Prevent blindness
    c. Restore the layers to their normal positions
    d. B and C

57. Scleral buckling is performed when the _____ of the retina becomes separated from the pigmented epithelial layer.
    a. Sensory layer
    b. Vascular layer
    c. Nervous layer
    d. Neurovascular bundle

58. Fragmentation of tissue by ultrasonic vibration is called _____.
    a. Scleral buckling
    b. Phacoemulsification
    c. Strabismus
    d. Penetrating keratoplasty

59. _____ is full-thickness transplantation of a donor cornea to restore vision.
    a. Scleral buckling
    b. Phacoemulsification
    c. Strabismus
    d. Penetrating keratoplasty

60. A condition in which the eye (or eyes) cannot focus on an object because the muscles lack coordination is called _____.
    a. Strabismus
    b. Pterygium
    c. Chalazion
    d. Entropion

61. The types of electrosurgical systems commonly used in eye surgery include the bipolar unit and the _____ unit.
    a. Handheld monopolar
    b. Single-use, battery powered
    c. Foot-activated monopolar
    d. Battery-powered bipolar

62. Shifting the patient immediately after surgery may result in _____ .
    a. Headache
    b. Pain
    c. Increased intraocular pressure and eye injury
    d. All of the above

63. A handheld instrument that magnifies the focal point, enabling the examiner to evaluate the fundus and other internal eye structures, is called _____.
    a. Magnifying glass
    b. Surgeon's loupes
    c. Operative microscope
    d. Ophthalmoscope

Case Study 1

Read the following case study and answer the questions based on your knowledge of the muscles of the eye.

To participate in an R&R (recession and resection) of the right eye, you must fully understand the musculature of the eye and how these muscles interact.

64. First, label the following picture.

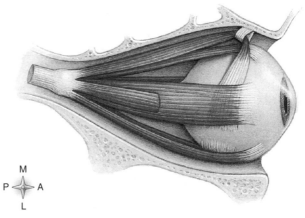

From Thibodeau G, Patton K: *Anatomy and physiology,* ed 6, St Louis, 2007, Mosby.

65. Now color-code the sets of muscles.

66. During an R&R, which muscle is resected?_____

67. Which muscle is regressed? _____

Case Study 2

You are about to scrub for a left cataract extraction with an IOL.

68. What is the protocol for implantation of an IOL?

_____

_____

_____

_____

The protocol includes:

(1) _____

_____

(2) _____

_____

(3) _____

_____

(4) _____

_____

INTERNET EXERCISES

Internet Exercise 1

Using your favorite search engine, type in the key words **penetrating keratoplasty** *and* **new advances.** *Read an article on advances in corneal transplantation and then answer the following questions.*

69. What Internet site did you find? _____

_____

70. What type of patient commonly undergoes this type of procedure? _____

_____

71. Why would a patient need this procedure? _____

_____

72. What would prevent a person from receiving a transplant? _____

_____

_____

73. Are surgical innovations being used in the procedure? _____

_____

_____

74. Are innovations being used in the tissue used for transplantation? _____

_____

75. Are innovations being used in the medications given to the perioperative patient?

_____

_____

_____

27 Surgery of the Ear, Nose, Pharynx, and Larynx

Student's Name _____

KEY TERMS

Write the definition for each term.

1. Canalplasty _____

2. Cerumen _____

3. Effusion _____

4. Evert _____

5. Goiter _____

6. Hypertrophy (hypertrophic) _____

7. Innervation _____

8. Keratin _____

9. Otitis media _____

10. Packing _____

11. Nasolaryngoscope _____

12. Neoplasm _____

13. Ossicles _____

14. Ototoxic _____

15. Packing _____

16. Paranasal sinus _____

17. Perforation _____

18. Perichondrium _____

19. Periosteum _____

20. Sublingual _____

21. TM _____

22. Transsphenoidal _____

23. Tympanostomy tube _____

24. Uvulopalatopharyngoplasty (UPP) _____

231

Provide a short answer for each question.

25. What is the specific anatomy of the larynx?

_____

_____

_____

_____

_____

26. What is the normal patient position for ENT procedures?

_____

_____

_____

_____

_____

LABELING

Label the structures of the ear.

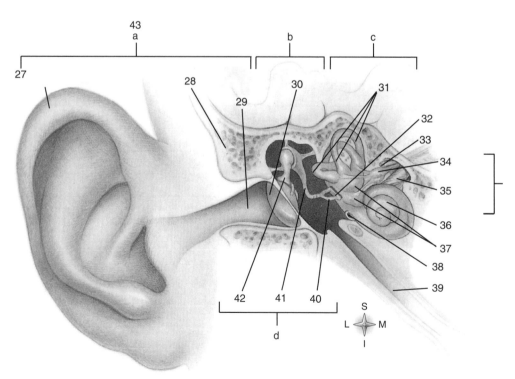

From Thibodeau G, Patton K: *Anatomy and physiology,* ed 6, St Louis, 2007, Mosby.

27. _____   35. _____

28. _____   36. _____

29. _____   37. _____

30. _____   38. _____

31. _____   39. _____

32. _____   40. _____

33. _____   41. _____

34. _____   42. _____

43. Now label the same drawing with the following:
    a. External ear
    b. Middle ear
    c. Inner ear
    d. Auditory ossicles

MATCHING

Match each term with the correct definition.

44. _____ A benign tumor of the middle ear caused by shedding of
            keratin in chronic otitis media

45. _____ Inability to maintain balance or the perception of spinning,
            falling, or the environment turning

46. _____ Drainage from the nose

47. _____ A benign epithelial tumor characterized by a branching
            or lobular shape

48. _____ Fluid in the middle ear

49. _____ Bleeding arising from the nasal cavity

50. _____ Vibration of the vocal cords during speaking or vocalization

51. _____ Rapid oscillation of the eye, symptomatic of certain diseases
            of the nervous system

52. _____ Paralysis of a structure, such as vocal cord paresis

53. _____ Excessive proliferation of mucosal epithelium

54. _____ Hearing impairment arising from the cochlea, auditory
            nerve, or central nervous system

55. _____ Abnormal thickening of the bone in the middle and
            inner ear

a. Cholesteatoma

b. Papilloma

c. Polyp

d. Vertigo

e. Epistaxis

f. Effusion

g. Rhinorrhea

h. Paresis

i. Sensorineural hearing loss

j. Nystagmus

k. Phonation

l. Otosclerosis

Indicate whether the statement is true or false.

56. The structures of the external ear include the outer surface of the tympanic membrane and all structures lateral to it.

_____ True   _____ False

57. The cochlea is round.

_____ True   _____ False

58. Infection of the middle ear may be acute or chronic.

_____ True   _____ False

59. Abnormal thickening of the bone in the middle and inner ear causes restriction of the stapes footplate and conductive hearing loss.

_____ True   _____ False

60. Hypothyroidism may be congenital or acquired.

_____ True   _____ False

61. The operating microscope is used in all procedures of the middle or inner ear.

_____ True   _____ False

62. Myringotomy is done to release fluid from the middle ear.

_____ True   _____ False

63. Tympanomastoidectomy is removal of soft tissue lining the mastoid cells.

_____ True   _____ False

64. Sound normally is received by the TM, which transmits vibration through the ossicles.

_____ True   _____ False

65. The semicircular canals communicate with the middle ear via the oval and round windows.

_____ True   _____ False

66. The cochlea contains the cochlear duct and organ of hearing.

_____ True   _____ False

67. The inner ear contains receptors for hearing and balance and is composed of a series of hollow tunnels called *labyrinths*.

_____ True   _____ False

68. The nose, oropharynx, and larynx share functions with the respiratory tract.

_____ True   _____ False

69. The neck is organized into triangles for study.

_____ True   _____ False

MULTIPLE CHOICE

Choose the most correct answer to complete the question or statement.

70. The membranous labyrinth is composed of three parts, including all of the following *except* the:
    a. Cochlea
    b. Tympanic membrane
    c. Semicircular canals
    d. Vestibule

71. The organ of hearing is called the _____.
    a. Organ of Corti
    b. Tympanic membrane
    c. Vestibule
    d. Cochlea

72. The _____ is (are) responsible for equilibrium of the body in motion.
    a. Organ of Corti
    b. Islets of Langerhans
    c. Crista ampullaris
    d. Otitis media

73. Medications used during ear surgery include all of the following *except* _____.
    a. Anesthetics
    b. Hemostatic agents
    c. Antibiotic solutions
    d. Viscoelastic agents

74. The thyroid secretes the hormones _____ .
    a. Thyroxin and triiodothyronine
    b. Thyroid-stimulating hormone (TSH) and triiodothyronine
    c. Iodine and thyroxin
    d. Parathyroid hormone and iodine

75. A _____ is a surgical opening made in the tympanic membrane.
    a. Myringotomy
    b. Myringectomy
    c. Iridectomy
    d. Stapedectomy

76. The most common cause of ossicle immobility is _____
    a. Stapedectomy
    b. Otosclerosis of the stapes
    c. Cancer
    d. Granuloma formation

77. During thyroplasty, the vocal cord is moved to one side and stabilized with a _____.
    a. Bridal suture
    b. Lahey thyroid retractor
    c. Green retractor
    d. Silastic or Gore-Tex implant

78. Surgery of the nose, oropharynx, and larynx is performed by a (an) _____.
    a. Optometrist
    b. Otorhinolaryngologist
    c. Dentist
    d. Doctor of osteopathy

79. The external nose is formed by two U-shaped cartilaginous structures called the _____
    a. Bilateral turbinates
    b. Nares
    c. Lower lateral cartilages
    d. Upper lateral cartilages

80. The _____ is (are) considered the floor of the nose.
    a. Palatine bone
    b. Paranasal sinuses
    c. Upper lateral cartilages
    d. Cribriform plate

235

81. The _____ separates the posterior aspect of the nasal cavities from the nasopharynx.
    a. Sinus
    b. Septum
    c. Ventricle
    d. Choana

82. The _____ lies at the posterosuperior extent of the nasal cavity.
    a. Vestibule
    b. Frontal sinus
    c. Sphenoid sinus
    d. Maxillary sinus

CASE STUDIES

Case Study 1

Read the following case study and answer the questions.

Choanal atresia is a congenital stricture of the choana that may require emergency surgery to restore respiration. Understanding the anatomy of the stricture is important to understanding the surgical procedure. Answer the following questions about choanal atresia.

83. What is the primary age group affected by the deformity? _____

84. What is the nature of the anomaly?

    _____

    _____

85. Explain the term *obligate nose breather*.

    _____

    _____

86. Describe the repair step by step.

    a. _____

    b. _____

    c. _____

    d. _____

    e. _____

    f. _____

Case Study 2

Read the following case study and answer the questions.

If you are about to scrub for a radical neck dissection, you will have to know the extent of the dissection or the degree of pathology.

What are the three types of neck dissection? What is involved in each?

87. _____

_____

_____

_____

88. _____

_____

_____

_____

89. _____

_____

_____

_____

INTERNET EXERCISES

Internet Exercise 1

Many of the cranial nerves are involved in the ENT procedures discussed in this chapter. Knowledge of the anatomy of the head and neck requires memorization of the 12 pairs of nerves that originate in the brain, each with a separate name and function. To help you learn the nerves and their functions, use your favorite search engine and type in the key term **medical mnemonics.** *Once you find a Web site, answer the following questions about the page.*

90. What Web page did you use?

_____

91. What acronym did you find to help you learn the names of the 12 pairs of cranial nerves?

_____

_____

92. Using the acronym that you found, list the 12 nerve pairs and their main function.

a. _____

b. _____

c. _____

d. _____

e. _____

f. _____

g. _____

h. _____

i. _____

j. _____

k. _____

l. _____

28 Oral and Maxillofacial Surgery

Student's Name _____

KEY TERMS

Write the definition for each term.

1. Arch bars _____

2. Bicoronal incision _____

3. Bicortical screw _____

4. Blowout fracture _____

5. Dentition _____

6. LeFort I fracture _____

7. LeFort II fracture _____

8. LeFort III fracture _____

9. Maxillomandibular fixation _____

10. Odontectomy _____

11. Transosteal implant _____

SHORT ANSWER

Provide a short answer for the question.

12. Procedures involving facial reconstruction and facial trauma involve a multidisciplinary team. Who are the members

   of this team? _____

   _____

   _____

Facial trauma may involve the many bones of the face and frontal sinus. To increase your knowledge of the anatomy of the bones of the face, label the following diagram.

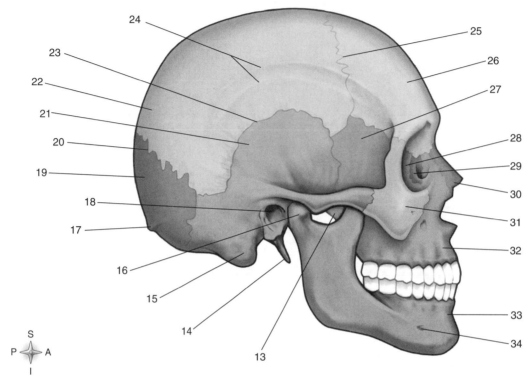

Modified from Thibodeau GA, Patt KT: *Anthony's textbook of anatomy and physiology,* ed 17, St Louis, 2003, Mosby.

13. _____   24. _____

14. _____   25. _____

15. _____   26. _____

16. _____   27. _____

17. _____   28. _____

18. _____   29. _____

19. _____   30. _____

20. _____   31. _____

21. _____   32. _____

22. _____   33. _____

23. _____   34. _____

To increase your knowledge of the anatomy of the bones of the face, label the following diagram.

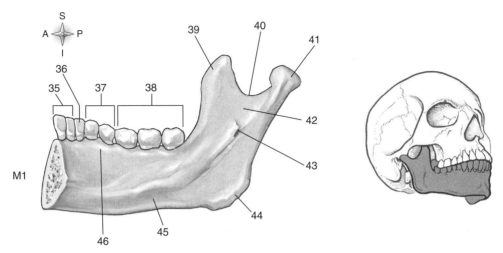

Modified from Thibodeau GA, Patt KT: *Anthony's textbook of anatomy and physiology,* ed 17, St Louis, 2003, Mosby.

35. _____   41. _____

36. _____   42. _____

37. _____   43. _____

38. _____   44. _____

39. _____   45. _____

40. _____   46. _____

MATCHING

Match each term with the correct definition.

47. _____ Realignment of the dentition of the mandible and midface

48. _____ Weight-bearing structures of the face

49. _____ Involved in "blow out" fractures

50. _____ Used to replace injured or lost dentition

51. _____ Knuckle-shaped portion of bone

52. _____ Open reduction and internal fixation of a fracture

53. _____ Procedure performed to remove teeth

a. Maxillomandibular fixation

b. ORIF

c. Buttresses

d. Condyle

e. Orbital floor

f. Frontal sinus

g. Dental implants

h. Odontectomy

TRUE/FALSE

Indicate whether the statement is true or false.

54. The frontal bone forms the upper part of the orbits.

_____ True   _____ False

55. The maxilla holds the palate and extends laterally to the zygoma and temporal bone.

_____ True   _____ False

56. Malar complex fractures often are called tripod and tetrapod fractures.

_____ True   _____ False

57. A dental implant is used only to replace multiple broken or missing teeth.

_____ True   _____ False

58. Supraperiosteal dental implants are placed beneath the periosteum directly on the alveolar bone.

_____ True   _____ False

59. Mandibular defects are congenital and usually are represented by a recessed mandible.

_____ True   _____ False

60. It is extremely important that wire cutters be sent with the patient, both to the recovery room and home, to allow release in case of an airway emergency.

_____ True   _____ False

MULTIPLE CHOICE

Choose the most correct answer to complete the question or statement.

61. Which of the following bones is shaped like a butterfly?
   a. Sphenoid bone
   b. Ethmoid bone
   c. Nasal bone
   d. Frontal bone

62. The teeth are embedded in the alveolus of the _____.
   a. Mandible
   b. Maxillary bones
   c. Ethmoid
   d. Mental foramen

63. The procedure performed to repair leakage of cerebral spinal fluid is called _____.
   a. ORIF mandible fracture
   b. ORIF orbital floor fractures
   c. La Forte osteotomy
   d. ORIF frontal sinus fracture

64. _____ is performed to reduce pain and increase mobility.
   a. ORIF
   b. La Forte osteotomy
   c. TMJ arthroplasty
   d. MMF

65. Which of the following procedures includes an implant?
   a. La Forte osteotomy
   b. TMJ arthroplasty
   c. MMF
   d. Closed reduction mandibular fracture

Case Study 1

66. Many diagrams of the midface, mandible, and other bony anatomy include a medical descriptive term, *process*. What does this term indicate with regard to bone? You may have to look this up in your medical terminology text.

_____

_____

_____

Case Study 2

Your patient has a malar complex fracture. You know that for the "complex" to be mobile, five fractures must be involved. Which "cheek" bones are involved in a malar complex fracture?

67. _____

68. _____

69. _____

70. _____

71. _____

INTERNET EXERCISES

Internet Exercise 1

*Using your favorite Internet search engine, type in the abbreviation **TMJ**. When you find a good medical site, answer the following questions.*

72. What Internet site did you use? _____

_____

73. What does TMJ stand for?

_____

74. What are the symptoms of TMJ?

_____

75. What nonsurgical interventions are used for someone suffering from TMJ?

_____

76. If someone has surgery for TMJ, what is the recovery time?

_____

29 Plastic and Reconstructive Surgery

Student's Name _____

KEY TERMS

Write the definition for each term.

1. Aesthetic surgery _____

2. Augment _____

3. Biological graft _____

4. Biosynthetic _____

5. Debridement _____

6. Eschar _____

7. Fasciotomy _____

8. Hydrodressing _____

9. Mohs surgery _____

10. Photodamage _____

11. Plication_____

12. Porcine _____

13. Ptosis _____

14. Stent _____

15. Undermine _____

SHORT ANSWERS

Provide a short answer to complete the question or statement.

16. Breast implants are made in different shapes and materials. Describe them and explain when they are used.

_____

_____

_____

17. Aside from age, what advances the aging process and what treatments are available to arrest the process?

_____

_____

_____

18. What are the specific goals of plastic surgery?

_____

_____

_____

19. What are the two fundamental types of grafts?

_____

_____

_____

20. What complications might a patient experience with liposuction?

_____

_____

_____

21. What are the five (5) epidermal layers that represent various developmental stages of the keratinocyte, and where is each layer primarily located?

a. _____

b. _____

c. _____

d. _____

e. _____

246

Label the following diagram of the epidermis, the structural layers of the skin.

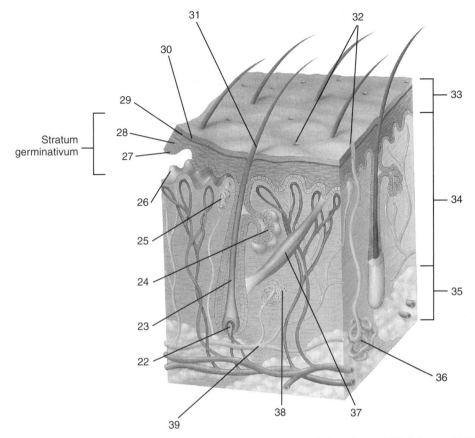

Stratum germinativum

Modified from Thibodeau GA, Patt KT: *Anthony's textbook of anatomy and physiology,* ed 17, St Louis, 2003, Mosby.

22. _____

23. _____

24. _____

25. _____

26. _____

27. _____

28. _____

29. _____

30. _____

31. _____

32. _____

33. _____

34. _____

35. _____

36. _____

37. _____

38. _____

39. _____

MATCHING

Match each term with the correct description.

40. _____ A graft transferred from one individual (human) to another

41. _____ A biological graft taken from one area of the body and transplanted to another area in the same patient

42. _____ A biological graft consisting of more than one tissue type

43. _____ A graft that contains only the dermis

44. _____ A graft derived from synthetic material compatible with body tissue. Synthetic grafts may be soft, semisolid, or liquid

45. _____ A graft containing the dermis and epidermis

46. _____ Tissue taken from one species and grafted to another

47. _____ A graft derived from live tissue, human or animal

a. Allograft

b. Full-thickness skin graft

c. Biological graft

d. Xenograft

e. Split-thickness skin graft

f. Composite graft

g. Autograft

h. Synthetic graft

TRUE/FALSE

Indicate whether the statement is true or false.

48. Panniculectomy is performed to remove excess skin and adipose tissue from the abdominal wall.

_____ True   _____ False

49. Liposuction instruments consist of rigid cannulas that are connected to a large-bore suction tube.

_____ True   _____ False

50. Liposuction is performed to remove excess superficial fat.

_____ True   _____ False

51. The TRAM flap can be used in a variety of plastic and reconstructive procedures.

_____ True   _____ False

52. Reduction mammoplasty is performed to increase the size of the breast tissue.

_____ True   _____ False

53. Preoperative preparation for breast surgery includes measurement and skin marking while the patient is standing to ensure a natural reconstruction.

_____ True   _____ False

54. Breast ptosis may be caused by breast feeding.

_____ True   _____ False

55. Facial augmentation is performed to correct underprojection of either the chin or the cheek.

_____ True   _____ False

56. Malignant lesions usually result from sun damage to the skin and include basal cell carcinoma.

_____ True   _____ False

MULTIPLE CHOICE

Choose the most correct answer to complete the question or statement.

57. After significant weight loss, the skin of the abdomen hangs flaccid and can interfere with movement by forming a(an) _____.
    a. Pannus
    b. Seroma
    c. Lipoma
    d. Emboli

58. Another name for panniculectomy is _____.
    a. Lipectomy
    b. Mastectomy
    c. Abdominoplasty
    d. Liposuction

59. _____ is performed to reconstruct the breast without the use of implants.
    a. Augmentation
    b. Mammoplasty
    c. Microtia
    d. A transverse rectus abdominis myocutaneous flap

60. The first step in the TRAM flap procedure is to _____.
    a. Remove the mastectomy scar
    b. Undermine the skin superior to the incision site
    c. Make an elliptical incision
    d. Ligate the inferior epigastric artery and vein

61. Macromastia is _____.
    a. Drooping breasts
    b. Excessively small breasts
    c. Excessively large breasts
    d. Nipple dysplasia

62. Micromastia in males is referred to as _____.
    a. Gynecomastia
    b. Male ptosis
    c. Benign tumors
    d. Enlarged nipples

63. Mastopexy is performed to correct _____.
    a. Lipomas
    b. Benign cystic breast disease
    c. Ductal cancer
    d. Breast ptosis

64. Cheiloplasty is _____.
    a. Cheek implants
    b. Lip augmentation
    c. Chin shaving
    d. Lip reduction

65. _____ is performed to increase the size and improve the shape of the breast.
    a. Mastopexy
    b. Augmentation mammoplasty
    c. Reduction mammoplasty
    d. Gynecomastia

66. Chin augmentation is called _____.
    a. Mammoplasty
    b. Cheiloplasty
    c. Mentoplasty
    d. Abdominoplasty

67. _____ is performed to rejuvenate an aging face, particularly the lower one third of the face, including the jaw line and neck.
    a. Liposuction
    b. Rhytidectomy
    c. Cheiloplasty
    d. Mentoplasty

68. This layer in the epidermis is relatively transparent and composed of dead keratinocytes that are filled with a protein called *keratin*.
    a. Stratum corneum
    b. Stratum lucidum
    c. Stratum granulosum
    d. Stratum germinativum

69. A skin graft can do all of the following *except:*
    a. Replace tissue that has been lost
    b. Augment (build up) tissue for aesthetic purposes
    c. Provide tissue for functional purposes
    d. Fill in a muscular defect

70. Macromastia can cause _____.
    a. Increased self-esteem
    b. Weight gain
    c. Lumbar back pain
    d. Cervical and thoracic pain

Case Study 1

Read the following case study and complete the exercise based on your knowledge of burns.

Your patient is coming to surgery for debridement of a burn. Your knowledge of burns helps you choose the skin grafting instruments that will be needed. Describe the different types of burns listed below using the American Burn Association classification system.

71. Superficial partial thickness first degree _____

_____

_____

72. Partial thickness second degree _____

_____

_____

73. Full thickness second degree _____

_____

_____

74. Full thickness third degree _____

_____

_____

Case Study 2

Your pediatric patient has microtia.

75. What is microtia? How would reconstruction be performed and at what age?

_____

_____

_____

_____

Internet Exercise 1

Using your favorite search engine, go to any plastic surgery site to research the pros and cons of Botox injections. Once you complete your research, answer the following questions.

76. What Internet site did you find? _____

77. What can the patient expect as far as the treatment is concerned? _____

_____

_____

78. How is the Botox administered? _____

_____

_____

79. Where are the procedures done? _____

_____

_____

80. Is there a recovery phase? _____

_____

_____

81. How long do the treatments last? _____

_____

_____

82. How much do the injections cost? _____

83. What medication is used in Botox injections? _____

84. What is the history of the drug? _____

_____

_____

85. How is the drug classified medically? _____

_____

_____

Internet Exercise 2

Your patient has come to surgery for a mastectomy for DCIS.

86. Go online and research this type of cancer. Then, offer a suggestion as to the type of mastectomy the patient will have to undergo.

_____

87. What are her reconstruction options after her mastectomy? _____

_____

_____

_____

88. If your patient is a cigarette smoker and her reconstruction requires a nipple reconstruction, what are the potential

complications for the graft as a result of the smoking? _____

_____

_____

_____

89. List your Internet site. _____

30 Orthopedic Surgery

Student's Name _____

KEY TERMS

Write the definition for each term.

1. Abduction _____

2. Adduction _____

3. Alloy _____

4. Aponeurosis _____

5. Arthrodesis _____

6. Arthroscopy _____

7. Biocompatibility _____

8. Biomechanics _____

9. Broach (broaching) _____

10. Cannulated _____

11. Casting _____

12. Comminuted _____

13. Debridement _____

14. Dislocation _____

15. External fixation _____

16. Fasciotomy _____

17. Inert _____

18. Internal fixation _____

19. Orthopedic system _____

20. Osteotomy _____

21. Ream _____

22. Replantation _____

23. Revision arthroplasty _____

24. Reduction _____

25. Slap hammer _____

26. Press-fit _____

Provide a short answer for each question or statement.

27. What are the three stages of bone healing, and what occurs during each phase? _____

    a. _____

    _____

    _____

    b. _____

    _____

    _____

    c. _____

    _____

    _____

28. How are joints classified?

    a. _____

    _____

    b. _____

    _____

    c. _____

    _____

    d. _____

    _____

    e. _____

    _____

For which of the following medical diagnoses would the surgical intervention be arthroplasty? If yes, write "yes" on the line; if no, write "no" on the line.

29. _____ Avascular necrosis

30. _____ Rheumatoid arthritis

31. _____ Malignant bone tumor

32. _____ Metastatic bone disease

33. _____ Osteoporosis

34. _____ Scoliosis

35. _____ Compartment syndrome

36. Define the fracture types listed below:

    a. Transverse _____

    b. Oblique _____

    c. Spiral _____

    d. Impacted _____

    e. Comminuted _____

    f. Open _____

    g. Greenstick _____

LABELING

Label this figure of the anatomy of a long bone using the descriptions and medical terminology as described in the text.

37. _____

38. _____

39. _____

40. _____

41. _____

42. _____

43. _____

44. _____

45. _____

46. _____

47. _____

48. _____

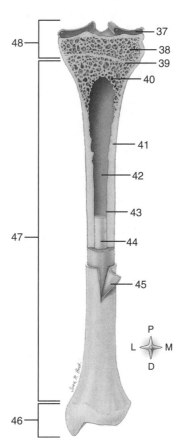

From Thibodeau G, Patton K: *Anatomy and physiology,* ed 6, St Louis, 2007, Mosby.

The figures below illustrate several types of orthopedic drills. Please label each illustration.

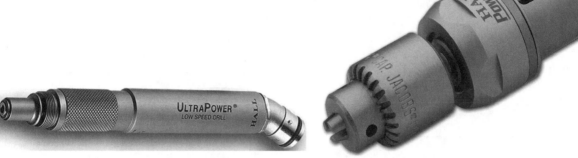

Courtesy Zimmer, Warsaw, Ind.

49. _____

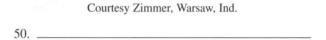

Courtesy Zimmer, Warsaw, Ind.

50. _____

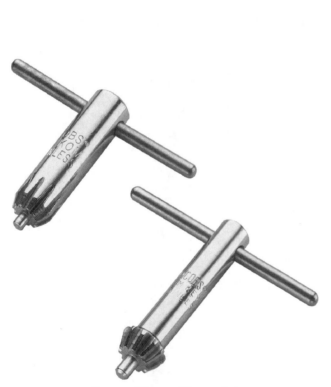

Courtesy Zimmer, Warsaw, Ind.

51. _____

Courtesy Zimmer, Warsaw, Ind.

52. _____

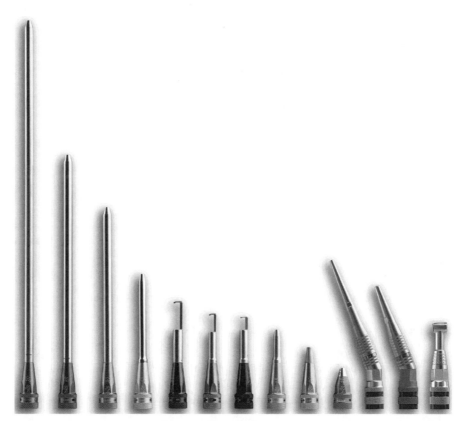

Courtesy Zimmer, Warsaw, Ind.

53. _____

Match each medical term for these bone landmarks with the correct definition.

54. _____ A ridge of bone

55. _____ A sharp, narrow projection

56. _____ A knuckle-shaped portion of bone, generally found in association with a joint

57. _____ A projection of bone

58. _____ A small, rounded projection

59. _____ A large, rounded projection

60. _____ A rounded orifice in bone, a passageway for blood vessels or nerves

61. _____ A cavity within a bone

62. _____ A groove in a bone

a. Sulcus

b. Crest

c. Condyle

d. Tubercle

e. Foramen

f. Sinus

g. Spine

h. Tuberosity

i. Process

Indicate whether the statement is true or false.

63. The *skeleton* provides structural support for the soft tissues of the body.

   _____ True   _____ False

64. The articular system includes those areas of the body where two bones meet and some degree of movement occurs.

   _____ True   _____ False

65. The orthopedic table is used mainly for surgery of the humerus and elbow.

   _____ True   _____ False

66. Bleeding bone commonly is controlled by using a compound made of paraffin wax.

   _____ True   _____ False

67. Open reduction of a fracture is performed by manipulation of the bone or with an external traction device.

   _____ True   _____ False

68. All power equipment used in surgery uses compressed nitrogen.

   _____ True   _____ False

69. Bioactive implants are absorbed by the body and stimulate or enhance bone repair.

   _____ True   _____ False

70. The Association for the Advancement of Medical Instrumentation (AAMI) institutes international protocols for patient safety when orthopedic implants are used.

   _____ True   _____ False

71. Orthopedic plates exert different forces on the fracture, the plate, and the soft tissue, depending on the type of plate.

   _____ True   _____ False

72. Bone graft substitutes are commonly used to repair and reconstruct bone and may be made from ceramic or polymer substances.

   _____ True   _____ False

73. *Biocompatibility* means that the implant is inert.

   _____ True   _____ False

74. The vapors released when the dry and liquid components of bone cement are mixed are known to cause serious eye damage, as well as respiratory tract and skin irritation.

_____ True   _____ False

MULTIPLE CHOICE

Choose the most correct answer to complete the question or statement.

75. Which of the following statements describes external fixation?
    a. The fracture is reduced manually or with a traction device and pinning.
    b. Reduction takes place through an incision as part of the surgery.
    c. Surgery and implants are required to hold bone fragments in place.
    d. The process is a means of stabilizing the bone from outside the body.

76. _____ remains the most common type of material used to make orthopedic implants.
    a. Plastic
    b. Polypropylene
    c. Stainless steel
    d. Titanium

77. Orthopedic screws are commonly used to do all of the following *except:*
    a. Attach a metal implant to bone
    b. Attach bone to bone
    c. Attach bone to soft tissue
    d. Repair defects in muscle such as the biceps

78. Which of the following is NOT a type of bone screw?
    a. Lag
    b. Herbert
    c. Cancellous
    d. Marrow

79. Which of the following statements is true with regard to compression screws?
    a. The screw thread applies compression only on the object furthest from the screw head.
    b. When tapping for this type of screw, the size of the drill tap is slightly smaller than the screw diameter.
    c. A glide hole technique is not used.
    d. The hole is drilled through both fragments.

80. IM nails are used for _____.
    a. Pelvic fractures
    b. Wrist fractures
    c. Fractures of long bones
    d. Intertrochanteric fractures

81. The main advantages of the K-wire and Steinmann pin include all of the following *except:*
    a. Their size
    b. Ease of insertion
    c. They cause little trauma to bone.
    d. They must be removed under general anesthesia.

82. The selection of implant material or design is based on _____.
    a. The patient's bone type
    b. The patient's age
    c. The patient's activity level
    d. All of the above

83. Which statement regarding the use of orthopedic bone cement is true?
    a. It is nonallergenic.
    b. It is a hazardous chemical and must be handled according to hospital policy protocol.
    c. It is nontoxic to the patient.
    d. It is associated with brain damage

Case Study 1

Read the following case study and answer the question.

Your patient has just arrived in the emergency department with orthopedic trauma. He will need to be evaluated and then diagnosed using a variety of imaging procedures. These commonly include which techniques?

84. _____

_____

85. _____

_____

86. _____

_____

87. _____

_____

88. _____

_____

Case Study 2

You have just been called in for orthopedic trauma. Knowing the types of bone fractures helps you choose the type of instrumentation needed for the repair. Working from left to right, label the fractures pictured in the following figure.

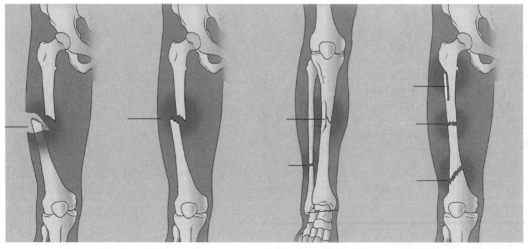

From Thibodeau G, Patton K: *Anatomy and physiology,* ed 6, St Louis, 2007, Mosby.

89. _____   93. _____

90. _____   94. _____

91. _____   95. _____

92. _____

INTERNET EXERCISES

Internet Exercise 1

Using your favorite search engine, look for medical mnemonics that will help you study the anatomy of bones. Choose some that will help you with this chapter and list them below.

96. What site did you use? _____

97. List one of the mnemonics you found. _____

_____

_____

_____

_____

Internet Exercise 2

Using your favorite search engine, find an orthopedic implant company. Look at the site as if you were a patient looking for information about your upcoming total knee arthroplasty. Then answer the following questions.

98. What site did you find? _____

99. What company did you find? _____

100. What "system" does the company use for the total knee? _____

_____

101. Are there pictures on the site of the instruments that will be used? If so, what are they?

_____

_____

102. Does the site include information about the procedure? _____

_____

103. Is there information for the patient about the postoperative recovery? _____

_____

_____

31 Peripheral Vascular Surgery

Student's Name _____

KEY TERMS

Write the definition for each term.

1. Angioplasty _____

2. Arteriotomy _____

3. Arteriovenous fistula _____

4. Bifurcation _____

5. Diastolic pressure _____

6. Doppler duplex ultrasonography _____

   _____

7. Electroencephalogram (EEG) _____

8. Embolus _____

9. Endarterectomy _____

10. Extracorporeal _____

11. Hemodialysis _____

12. Hemodynamic _____

13. Infarction _____

14. In situ _____

15. Intravascular ultrasound _____

16. Lumen _____

17. Percutaneous _____

18. Stasis _____

19. Stent _____

20. Systolic pressure _____

21. Thrombus _____

22. Vessel loop _____

Label the pulmonary and systemic vascular circulation.

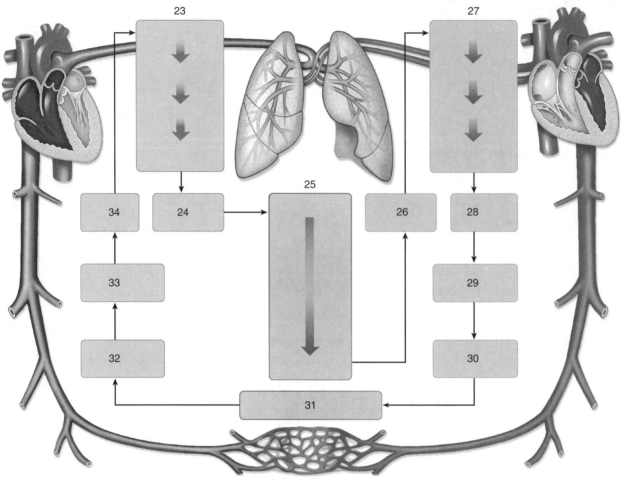

Modified from Thibodeau G, Patton K: *Anatomy and physiology,* ed 6, St Louis, 2007, Mosby.

23. _____

24. _____

25. _____

26. _____

27. _____

28. _____

29. _____

30. _____

31. _____

32. _____

33. _____

34. _____

Working from left to right, label the vascular clamps shown.

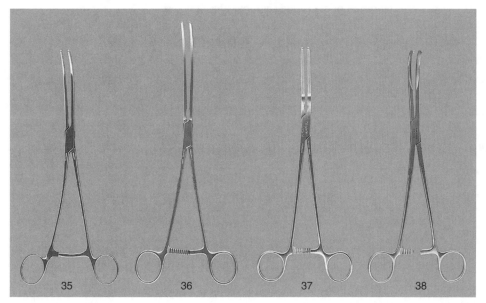

From Tighe SM: *Instrumentation for the operating room,* ed 7, St Louis, 2007, Mosby.

35. _____

36. _____

37. _____

38. _____

MATCHING

Match each disease process with the correct definition.

39. _____ Ballooning or dilation of an artery caused by stricture and increased arterial pressure

40. _____ Clot of blood, air, or organic material that moves freely in the vascular system

41. _____ Drop in blood pressure related to reduced vascular volume

42. _____ Abnormal increase in blood pressure

43. _____ Blockage in an artery, leading to ischemia and tissue death

44. _____ Voluntary action in which air is forced against a closed glottis

45. _____ The most common form of arteriosclerosis, which causes plaque to form on the inner surface of an artery

46. _____ Lack of blood and therefore oxygen in tissue

47. _____ Abnormal lowering of blood pressure

48. _____ Disease characterized by thickening, hardening, and loss of elasticity of the artery walls

a. Aneurysm

b. Arteriosclerosis

c. Atherosclerosis

d. Embolus

e. Hypotension

f. Hypovolemia

g. Hypertension

h. Infarction

i. Ischemia

j. Valsalva

Indicate whether the statement is true or false.

49. The lymphatic system is composed of ducts and regional lymph nodes.

  _____ True   _____ False

50. Blood pressure is the force that is exerted on the arterial wall by the pumping action of the heart.

  _____ True   _____ False

51. The most commonly used vessel dissection scissors are Potts scissors.

  _____ True   _____ False

52. Venous blood is bright red.

  _____ True   _____ False

53. When severed, arteries tend to spurt blood because it is under pressure from the pumping of the heart.

  _____ True   _____ False

54. Both veins and arteries are composed of multiple tissue layers or walls.

  _____ True   _____ False

55. Lack of exercise causes venous stasis or pooling of blood in the veins.

  _____ True   _____ False

56. A Z-shaped vessel is called a *bifurcation*.

  _____ True   _____ False

57. The popliteal artery is an extension of the femoral artery.

  _____ True   _____ False

58. Nodes collect and filter fluid from the lymph ducts and are the site of lymphocyte production.

  _____ True   _____ False

59. Lymph vessels follow the anatomical pattern of arteries and veins.

  _____ True   _____ False

60. Vascular surgery requires a number of important and potentially harmful intraoperative drugs.

  _____ True   _____ False

61. Before the carotid arteriotomy is closed, the external, internal, and common carotid artery clamps are opened and closed, in that order.

_____ True   _____ False

MULTIPLE CHOICE

Choose the most correct answer to complete the question or statement.

62. Which of the following statements is false with regard to arteries?
    a. Arteries have thicker walls than do veins.
    b. Arteries must withstand pressure created by the heart contraction.
    c. Arteries are more elastic than veins.
    d. Arteries have interior valves.

63. Synthetic vascular grafts are made of all the following *except* _____.
    a. Dacron
    b. Polyester
    c. Nylon
    d. Gore-Tex

64. All of the following are used in vessel retraction *except* _____.
    a. Penrose drains
    b. Silastic loops
    c. Umbilical tapes
    d. Fogarty catheters

65. A _____ is a small metal implant designed to fit against the wall of an artery.
    a. Vascular stent
    b. Vascular bolster
    c. Rubber bolster
    d. Vascular catheter

66. Vascular stents are made of _____.
    a. Stainless steel
    b. Dacron
    c. Titanium
    d. Metal alloy

67. Heparinized saline solution is:
    a. Used to soak Gelfoam, which is placed on a grafted suture line
    b. Administered before the blood vessels are exposed
    c. Used to irrigate open vessels
    d. Administered with protamine sulfate

68. A dry power that is reconstituted with saline is _____.
    a. Heparin sulfate
    b. Protamine sulfate
    c. Topical thrombin
    d. Gelfoam

69. _____ may be injected into the vessel to prevent vasospasm during surgery.
    a. Heparin
    b. Lidocaine
    c. Thrombin
    d. Marcaine

70. Intraoperative angiography is used in conjunction with _____.
    a. Angioplasty
    b. Thrombectomy
    c. Anastomosis
    d. Graft placement

71. Thrombus is:
    a. A blood clot in the arterial or venous system
    b. A blood clot that is moving through the venous system
    c. Another name for a heart attack
    d. Remodeling of the shape of the artery

72. Hemodialysis is necessary for survival when the kidneys' filtering ability drops below _____.
    a. 2%
    b. 5%
    c. 7%
    d. 10%

73. Arteriovenous fistula is:
    a. A graft placed between an artery and a vein
    b. An abnormal tunnel that forms between a vein and an artery
    c. The remodeling of a vein or an artery without the use of a stent
    d. A direct anastomosis between an artery and a vein

Case Study 1

Read the following case study and answer the question based on your knowledge of the physiology of blood pressure.

Assessment of a patient's blood pressure is a basic skill that must be mastered by nursing and allied health professionals. What factors can affect a patient's blood pressure reading?

74. _____

_____

75. _____

_____

76. _____

_____

77. _____

_____

78. _____

_____

79. _____

_____

80. _____

_____

81. _____

_____

82. _____

_____

83. _____

_____

Case Study 2

Patients with end-stage renal disease require frequent hemodialysis. This treatment requires long-term access to the patient's vascular system.

84. What surgical interventions might be needed to create a means of long-term access?

_____

_____

_____

_____

_____

_____

_____

_____

_____

INTERNET EXERCISES

Internet Exercise 1

Using your favorite search engine, find some Web sites written for health care professionals that describe peripheral artery disease (PAD). After researching a couple of sites, pick one with good information and answer the following questions.

85. What Web site did you find that had good information on the disease process?

_____

_____

86. What did you learn about the effects of smoking on the peripheral vascular system?

_____

_____

_____

87. Which peripheral vascular diseases are directly linked to smoking?

_____

_____

_____

The United States has many excellent heart institutes. Using your favorite search engine, find three hospitals close to your home that deal with vascular and heart disease.

88. What are their names and where are they located?

1. _____

2. _____

3. _____

89. Go to the Web site for the Texas Heart Institute (THI) in Houston. Look for continued education events. What did you find there?

_____

_____

_____

90. Does THI offer continuing education courses that would provide appropriate continuing education units (CEUs) for you as a graduate surgical technologist? If so, name two or three of them.

_____

_____

91. On the THI Web site, search for Dr. Denton Cooley. Who is he?

_____

_____

_____

92. Also on the THI Web site, search for Dr. Michael DeBakey. Who was he?

_____

_____

_____

93. Does the Web site offer information for patients and other individuals who are not health care professionals? If so, give two or three examples.

_____

_____

32 Thoracic and Pulmonary Surgery

Student's Name _____

KEY TERMS

Write the definition for each term.

1. Arterial blood gases _____

2. Blebs _____

3. Closed chest drainage _____

4. Diffusion _____

5. Dyspnea _____

6. Empyema _____

7. Expiration _____

8. Hemoptysis _____

9. Hemothorax _____

10. Inspiration _____

11. Perfusion _____

12. Pleur-Evac _____

13. Pneumothorax _____

14. Pulmonary function tests _____

15. Thoracoscopy _____

16. Thoracotomy _____

17. Ventilation _____

SHORT ANSWERS

Provide a short answer for each question or statement.

18. What organs and structures are located in the mediastinal space?

_____

_____

_____

19. Explain the pleural cavity. Include in your explanation the pleural sac, pleural space, and negative pressure.

_____

_____

_____

_____

20. What diagnostic tests would be done on a patient who will undergo lung and respiratory surgical procedures?

_____

_____

_____

_____

21. Explain the difference between bronchial washings, cytology brushing, and tissue biopsy.

_____

_____

_____

22. What is the difference between pneumonectomy, segmental resection, and wedge resection?

_____

_____

_____

_____

_____

_____

23. What type of pathology is involved in thoracic outlet syndrome? _____

_____

_____

_____

24. What procedure is performed to relieve thoracic outlet syndrome? _____

_____

Label the following diagram of a Pleur-Evac disposable chest suction system.

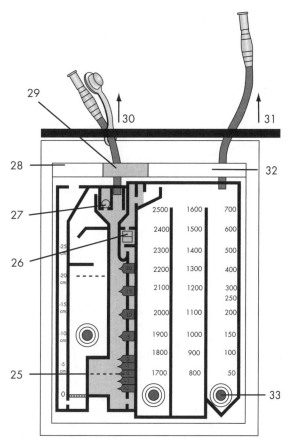

From Lewis SM, Heitkemper MM, Dirksen SR: *Medical-surgical nursing: assessment and management of clinical problems,* ed 6, St Louis, 2004, Mosby.

25. _____

26. _____

27. _____

28. _____

29. _____

30. _____

31. _____

32. _____

33. _____

34. Draw a diagram of the bilateral lungs. Be sure to label your drawing.

MATCHING

Match the medical diagnosis with the correct surgical intervention.

35. _____ Decortication of the lung

36. _____ Thymectomy

37. _____ Repair of pectus excavatum

38. _____ Lung transplantation

39. _____ Lung volume reduction

40. _____ Decortication of the lung

41. _____ Chest tube insertion for bleeding

42. _____ Chest tube insertion for spontaneous collapse lung

43. _____ Lobectomy

44. _____ Lung transplantation as a result of cigarette smoking, asthma, tuberculosis, and age-related atrophy

45. _____ Bronchoscopy

46. _____ Rib resection

a. Atelectasis

b. Bronchitis

c. Bone malformations

d. Cancer

e. Emphysema

f. Fibrosis

g. Hemothorax

h. Infectious diseases

i. Obstructive pulmonary disease

j. Pneumothorax

k. Myasthenia gravis

l. Thoracic outlet syndrome

m. Scarring from inflammation

TRUE/FALSE

Indicate whether the statement is true or false.

47. Video-assisted thoracoscopic surgery (VATS) is a minimally invasive technique for surgical procedures of the thoracic cavity.

_____ True   _____ False

48. Patients with lung cancer benefit from resection of portions of lung tissue that have been destroyed by the disease and are overinflated.

_____ True   _____ False

49. Flexible bronchoscopy generally is used only for removal of a large amount of tissue or a foreign body.

_____ True   _____ False

50. Flexible bronchoscopy is used to examine the lower respiratory tract and to obtain biopsy specimens.

_____ True   _____ False

51. Accessory instruments used with the flexible bronchoscope are smaller than those used with the rigid scope.

_____ True   _____ False

52. The goal of open chest drainage is to prevent the thorax from filling with air and thus deflating the lungs.

_____ True   _____ False

53. Negative pressure in the thoracic cavity is lost when the body wall and pleura are opened.

_____ True   _____ False

54. Lung biopsy most often is performed when other diagnostic tests, such as CT scans, bronchoscopy, and radiographs, do not reveal the cause of lung disease.

_____ True   _____ False

55. To inspect the lung during LVRS, the anesthesia care provider inflates and deflates areas of the pulmonary tissue.

_____ True   _____ False

56. The lumen of a rigid bronchoscope is larger than that of a flexible bronchoscope.

_____ True   _____ False

57. An important complication of rigid bronchoscopy is injury to the tracheobronchial structures.

_____ True   _____ False

58. A rigid bronchoscope has video capability, and the digital images are projected onto a video screen.

_____ True   _____ False

59. Thoracic outlet syndrome is a condition characterized by compression of the subclavian vessels and the brachial plexus at the apex of the thorax.

_____ True   _____ False

MULTIPLE CHOICE

Choose the most correct answer to complete the question or statement.

60. When patients are placed in the lateral position, an axillary roll is positioned to _____.
   a. Prevent pressure on the axillary nerves and blood vessels
   b. Facilitate heart function
   c. Reduce blood pressure
   d. Reduce the amount of bleeding

61. Lung biopsy is performed most often when _____.
   a. A CT scan indicates that the patient may have cancer.
   b. Bronchoscopy washings show that the patient has tuberculosis.
   c. Radiographs do not reveal the cause of lung disease.
   d. A previous percutaneous biopsy has indicated pulmonary fibrosis.

275

62. _____ is the insertion of a fiberoptic or rigid telescope into the trachea and bronchi to determine a diagnosis or for surgical intervention.
   a. Bronchotomy
   b. Bronchectomy
   c. Laryngotomy
   d. Bronchoscopy

63. Which of the following is an attachment to the suction?
   a. Duval
   b. Cytology brush
   c. Lukens trap
   d. Pennington

64. A major risk with flexible bronchoscopy that is not a factor with rigid bronchoscopy is:
   a. With rigid bronchoscopy, the patient cannot be ventilated through the tube.
   b. With flexible bronchoscopy, the patient must breathe around the flexible endoscope.
   c. With rigid bronchoscopy, the surgeon cannot take a biopsy sample.
   d. Flexible bronchoscopy can be used only in the superficial respiratory tract.

65. The surgeon obtains cytology samples by _____.
   a. Taking a wedge biopsy sample through VATS
   b. Inserting a biopsy "biter" through the rigid bronchoscopy
   c. Inserting a small brush through the operating channel of the flexible bronchoscope
   d. Collecting fluid through washings

66. In mediastinoscopy, the surgeon makes a(an) _____.
   a. Incision in the suprasternal notch
   b. Midline thoracic incision
   c. Combined thoracoabdominal incision
   d. Lateral thoracic incision

67. A potential complication in mediastinoscopy is:
   a. The lymphatic tissue and the aorta are difficult to tell apart.
   b. The patient will need two chest tubes after the procedure.
   c. The incision is made right over the heart, and the heart could be injured during the procedure.
   d. Major arteries and veins of the thoracic cavity lie close to the area being visualized and can be injured.

68. Which of the following statements describes pectus excavatum?
   a. In addition to the chest instruments, the surgeon may need plastic surgical instruments.
   b. Deformity of the costal cartilages causes a concave deformity of the sternum.
   c. The procedure is done through a lateral incision.
   d. Deformity of the sternum causes a convex deformity of the sternum.

69. In what position is the patient placed for a pneumonectomy?
   a. Supine
   b. Prone
   c. Fowler's position
   d. Lateral position

CASE STUDIES

Case Study 1

Read the following case study and answer the questions based on your knowledge of lung transplantation.

Your patient has a lung disease and will have to undergo lung transplantation. Answer the following questions about your patient and the procedure to better understand the operation.

70. What disease processes might precipitate the patient's need for a transplant?

_____

_____

71. In what position will your surgical patient be placed for the procedure?

_____

_____

72. Will your patient need to go on bypass for the procedure?

_____

_____

Case Study 2

73. Why is a local anesthetic sprayed into the trachea (even if the patient is under general anesthesia) before the endoscope is inserted for a bronchoscopy?

_____

_____

_____

INTERNET EXERCISES

Internet Exercise 1

Using your favorite search engine, look for the organ procurement organization that is closest to where you live. Once you find the Web site, answer the following questions about organ donation.

74. What is the name of the organ procurement organization closest to you?

_____

75. Where is it located? _____

76. How far from your location is it? _____

77. What are the qualifications for becoming a donor? _____

_____

_____

78. What are the qualifications for becoming a living donor? _____

_____

_____

79. What organs are used in living (familial) donation? _____

_____

_____

_____

33 Cardiac Surgery

Student's Name _____

KEY TERMS

Write the definition for each term.

1. Aneurysm _____
2. Apex _____
3. Arrhythmia _____
4. Arteriosclerosis _____
5. Bradycardia _____
6. Cardioplegia _____
7. Coarctation _____
8. Congenital _____
9. Cross-clamp _____
10. Endovascular repair _____
11. Fibrillation _____
12. Fusiform aneurysm _____
13. Heart lung machine _____
14. Infarction _____
15. Ischemia _____
16. Mediastinum _____
17. Off-pump procedure _____
18. Pacemaker _____
19. Preclotting _____
20. Saccular aneurysm _____
21. Shunt _____
22. Stenosis _____
23. Sternotomy _____
24. Systole _____
25. Tachycardia _____
26. Thoracotomy _____

SHORT ANSWER

Provide a short answer for the following question.

27. What structures are in the thoracic cavity? _____

_____

_____

LABELING

Using the following diagram, label the components of the conduction system of the heart.

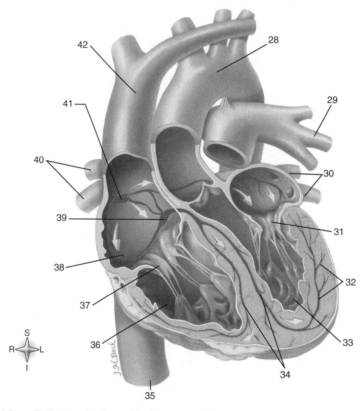

Modified from Thibodeau G, Patton K: *Anatomy and physiology,* ed 6, St Louis, 2007, Mosby.

28. _____   36. _____

29. _____   37. _____

30. _____   38. _____

31. _____   39. _____

32. _____   40. _____

33. _____   41. _____

34. _____   42. _____

35. _____

MATCHING

Match each term with the correct definition.

43. _____ Cancerous tumors

44. _____ Cause of CAD

45. _____ Condition in which the heart cells quiver rather than contract effectively

46. _____ Type of hardening of the arteries that results in stiffness and loss of function

47. _____ Weakening of the wall of an artery or the heart chamber, leading to thinning and ballooning

48. _____ Condition in which the heart is unable to eject a sufficient amount of blood to perfuse the body's tissues

49. _____ Excess fluid in the pericardium

50. _____ Chronic inflammation of the pericardium

51. _____ Heart rate below 60 beats per minute

52. _____ Possible narrowing of aortic and mitral valve or valves

53. _____ Cardiac muscle that beats abnormally fast

54. _____ Immune-mediated disease

a. Aneurysm
b. Atherosclerosis
c. Atrial fibrillation
d. Bradycardia
e. Congestive heart failure
f. Atherosclerosis
g. Neoplasm
h. Paracardial effusion
i. Pericarditis
j. Rheumatic heart disease
k. Valve stenosis
l. Tachycardia

TRUE/FALSE

Indicate whether the statement is true or false.

55. The valves of the heart maintain unidirectional blood flow.

_____ True   _____ False

56. The cardiac cycle is the pumping action from one beat to the next.

_____ True   _____ False

57. Cardiac catheterization is an interventional radiological procedure.

_____ True   _____ False

58. Left heart catheterization is performed through an incision into the femoral, radial, or brachial artery.

_____ True   _____ False

59. Cardiac instrumentation and procedures are quite routine, and beginning surgical technologists can easily anticipate the steps of a procedure.

_____ True   _____ False

60. A Rumel tourniquet is a complex component of cardiac instrumentation made partly from rubber tubing.

_____ True   _____ False

61. Prosthetic grafts are used to replace injured segments of an artery or a vein that is not affected by disease.

_____ True   _____ False

62. A pacemaker is a device that produces electrical impulses that stimulate the heart muscle.

_____ True   _____ False

63. Cardioplegia solution is the intentional interruption of the heart's pumping action.

_____ True   _____ False

64. The heart-lung machine takes the place of the heart and lungs by pumping and perfusing blood.

_____ True   _____ False

65. Procedures of the heart and associated structures are performed with the patient in the supine or lateral position with the affected side up.

_____ True   _____ False

MULTIPLE CHOICE

Choose the most correct answer to complete the question or statement.

66. Which of the following is NOT a heart valve?
    a. Atrial valve
    b. Mitral valve
    c. Tricuspid valve
    d. Cardiac valve

67. Which of the following are risk factors for atherosclerosis?
    a. Hypercholesterolemia
    b. Exercise
    c. Alcohol consumption
    d. Vegetarianism

68. A partial or full midline incision that is made through the sternum is called _____.
    a. Median sternotomy
    b. Paramedian
    c. Posterolateral
    d. Minithoracotomy

69. A 2-inch right or left incision made between the ribs for access during minimally invasive and robotic procedures is called a _____.
    a. Median sternotomy
    b. Paramedian
    c. Posterolateral
    d. Minithoracotomy

70. Cardiac surgery requires cardiac instruments and _____.
    a. General surgery instruments
    b. Orthopedic equipment
    c. Specialized skin closure
    d. Special laser equipment

71. Which of the following are common anticoagulants used intraoperatively? (Select all that apply.)
    a. Heparin sodium
    b. Protamine sulfate
    c. Topical thrombin
    d. Gelfoam

72. The heart-lung pump does all of the following *except:*
    a. Collects the blood and returns it to the body
    b. Removes excess carbon dioxide from the blood
    c. Changes the pH of the blood
    d. Oxygenates the blood

73. A _____ is a midline incision used for surgical procedures of the heart and great vessels in the thoracic cavity.
    a. Thoracoabdominal incision
    b. Paramedian incision
    c. Median sternotomy
    d. Costal incision

74. A cardioplegic solution is used to stop the heart:
    a. To reduce the energy required by the cardiac muscle by eliminating the energy requirements of contraction
    b. By increasing the energy required by the cardiac muscle, causing a cardiac arrest
    c. Only for external heart procedures
    d. Only for 20-minute increments

75. Which of the following are potential postoperative complications of bypass canalization? (Select all that apply.)
    a. Temporary cognitive, sensory, and perceptual changes in the patient
    b. Atelectasis
    c. Hemorrhage
    d. All of the above

76. Which of the following procedures requires a straight or bifurcated tube graft?
    a. Aortic aneurysmectomy
    b. Tetralogy of Fallot
    c. Mitral valve replacement
    d. CABG with IMA graft

CASE STUDIES

Case Study 1

77. Your patient has just had a heart attack and is asking about the term *cardiac cycle*. How would you explain the cardiac cycle to your patient?

    _____

    _____

    _____

INTERNET EXERCISES

Internet Exercise 1

Using your favorite search engine, search for cardiac transplantation procedures, particularly domino transplantation. After reading the information on this type of procedure, answer the following questions.

78. On what Web page did you find information?

    _____

79. What type of patient undergoes domino procedures? _____

    _____

    _____

80. How are the procedures different from normal cardiac transplantation? _____

    _____

    _____

    _____

Chapter **33 Cardiac Surgery**

Internet Exercise 2

Using your favorite search engine, do some research on the following pioneers of cardiac surgery. For each, give the date of birth and date of death. List the significant contributions each made to the field of cardiac surgery, transplantation, and antirejection drugs.

81. Walt Lillehi _____

_____

_____

_____

_____

82. Denton Cooley _____

_____

_____

_____

_____

83. Michael DeBakey _____

_____

_____

_____

_____

34 Pediatric Surgery

Student's Name _____

KEY TERMS

Write the definition for each term.

1. Acquired anomaly (defect) _____
2. Child life specialist _____
3. Choanal _____
4. Congenital _____
5. Ductus arteriosus _____
6. Genetic abnormality _____
7. Homeostasis _____
8. Isolette _____
9. Magical thinking _____
10. Mutagenic substance _____
11. Nephroblastoma _____
12. Prewarming _____
13. Teratogen _____
14. Thyroglossal duct _____

SHORT ANSWERS

Provide a short answer for each question or statement.

15. Name three interventions used to keep pediatric patients warm in surgery.

   a. _____

   b. _____

   c. _____

16. What is the surgical technologist's responsibility in reporting and calculating blood loss in pediatric patients?

   _____

   _____

   _____

17. Babies with esophageal atresia or a transesophageal fistula usually are low-birth-weight babies. Why? _____

_____

_____

_____

18. What is Hirschsprung's disease?

_____

_____

19. What is the difference between hypospadias and epispadias?

_____

_____

_____

_____

20. Coarctation of the thoracic aorta is a congenital stenosis. What does correction of this congenital condition do for

the patient?_____

_____

_____

_____

21. If your patient needs a pulmonary valvulotomy, what is the diagnosis? _____

_____

22. What are the specific defects in tetralogy of Fallot? _____

_____

_____

Match each medical diagnosis with the correct definition.

23. _____ Absence or closure of an orifice or a tubular structure

24. _____ Narrowing of the passageway of a blood vessel, such as coarctation of the aorta

25. _____ Eversion or turning out of an organ

26. _____ Herniation of abdominal contents through the abdominal wall, present at birth

27. _____ Telescoping of one portion of the intestine into another

28. _____ Wilms' tumor

29. _____ Congenital abnormality resulting from failure of the neural tube to close in embryonic development

30. _____ Protrusion of abdominal contents through an opening at the navel, especially when occurring as a congenital defect

31. _____ Narrowing of the part of the stomach (pylorus) that leads to the small intestines

a. Pyloric stenosis
b. Exstrophy
c. Coarctation
d. Atresia
e. Omphalocele
f. Neural tube defect
g. Gastroschisis
h. Nephroblastoma
i. Intussusception

TRUE/FALSE

Indicate whether the statement is true or false.

32. Pediatrics is the branch of medicine involved in the care of the child from the neonatal period to late adolescence.

_____ True   _____ False

33. Much of pediatric surgery is performed to correct physical defects that develop during fetal life.

_____ True   _____ False

34. Pediatric patients, especially adolescents, are particularly vulnerable to hypothermia.

_____ True   _____ False

35. Hypothermia can result in a chain of physiological events that put the pediatric patient at risk for cardiac problems, apnea, and hypoglycemia.

_____ True   _____ False

36. Infants lack the mechanism for shivering.

_____ True   _____ False

37. Physiological hyperthermia, such as malignant hyperthermia, is a greater risk in pediatric patients than in adults.

_____ True   _____ False

38. The body-to-surface-area ratio in infants and young children contributes to an increased risk for acid-base imbalance in the blood.

_____ True   _____ False

39. Bleeding is of no greater concern in pediatric patients than in any other patient.

_____ True   _____ False

40. Failure to manage the pediatric patient's airway is among the leading causes of death in medical and traumatic emergencies.

_____ True   _____ False

41. The safety principles that apply to adult electrosurgery are too high for pediatrics.

_____ True   _____ False

42. Although cleft palate sometimes is seen in conjunction with cleft lip, the two are separate malformations and are rarely related to one another.

_____ True   _____ False

43. Choanal atresia is a congenital anomaly.

_____ True   _____ False

MULTIPLE CHOICE

Choose the most correct answer to complete the question or statement.

44. The primary symptom of tetralogy of Fallot is _____.
    a. Shortness of breath
    b. Embolism
    c. Cyanosis
    d. Ischemia

45. The acronym for a hole in the interatrial septum is _____.
    a. PVC
    b. ASD
    c. PAC
    d. VSD

46. Which of the following statements is true regarding pulmonary valvulotomy?
    a. The pericardial sac is incised with scissors.
    b. The surgeon enters the chest through a median sternotomy.
    c. A purse-string suture of 4-0 polypropylene or polyester is placed around the aorta.
    d. Cardiopulmonary bypass is not needed.

47. An environmental agent that can injure the embryo or fetus is a _____ substance.
    a. Pediatric
    b. Congenital
    c. Mutagenic
    d. Teratogen

48. Which statement about thermoregulation is false?
    a. Physiological mechanisms that normally regulate temperature in an adult are absent or undeveloped in the infant.
    b. Children and infants have an extensive peripheral circulation, which contributes to relatively rapid cooling.
    c. Infants lack adequate surface area to maintain core temperature in a cold environment.
    d. Infants and children show a wide range in temperature variation compared to adults.

49. The _____ is the groove that extends from the upper lip to the nose.
    a. Philtrum
    b. Antrum
    c. Ventricle
    d. Septum

50. The term *branchial* refers to _____
    a. Gills
    b. Axilla
    c. Vessels
    d. Arm

51. _____ is surgery to correct infantile hypertrophic pyloric stenosis.
    a. Pylorosis
    b. Pyloromyotomy
    c. Pylorotomy
    d. Pyloroplasty

52. _____ a nongenetic defect in which the esophagus is interrupted.
    a. Esophageal atresia
    b. Esophagitis
    c. Esophagotomy
    d. Esophageal infection

53. _____ is characterized by a congenital absence of ganglion cells, which control the relaxation and contraction that occur in peristalsis.
    a. Omphalocele
    b. Gastroschisis
    c. Hirschsprung's disease
    d. Volvulus

54. _____ is the telescoping of one portion of the intestine into another.
    a. Intussusception
    b. Gastroschisis
    c. Hirschsprung's disease
    d. Volvulus

55. Reduction of a volvulus is performed to relieve intestinal obstruction by _____ of the affected bowel.
    a. Resection
    b. Stretching
    c. Untwisting
    d. Pulling

56. The most common malignant renal tumor in children is _____.
    a. Nephroma
    b. Cystoma
    c. Neuroblastoma
    d. Lipoma

CASE STUDIES

Case Study 1

Read the following case study and answer the questions

57. Some things both in the environment and in the diet of a pregnant woman are teratogenic to the fetus. What are they?

    _____

    _____

    _____

    _____

    _____

    _____

Case Study 2

Read the following case study and answer the questions.

58. Your patient has just been diagnosed with patent ductus. How is the patient's circulation abnormal? Was this child's circulatory pattern ever normal?

_____

_____

_____

_____

_____

_____

_____

INTERNET EXERCISES

Internet Exercise 1

Using your favorite search engine, search for several pediatric birth defects. When you find a site where you can research several defects at once, answer the following questions.

59. What Web site did you find? _____

60. How many of the pediatric birth defects occur as a single anomaly?

_____

_____

61. Do birth defects occur more often with premature infants? _____

_____

_____

Internet Exercise 2

Pectus excavatum does not have a genetic component, but it may be associated with Marfan's syndrome. Go online and explore Marfan's syndrome and then answer the following questions:

62. What Web site did you use? _____

63. What is Marfan's syndrome? _____

64. Are other defects associated with Marfan's syndrome? If so, what are they? _____

_____

_____

_____

_____

65. Is Marfan's syndrome hereditary? _____

66. Several famous people in history have had Marfan's syndrome. Name four of them.

    (1) _____

    (2) _____

    (3) _____

    (4) _____

35 Neurosurgery

Student's Name _____

KEY TERMS

Write the definition for each term.

1. Acoustic neuroma _____

2. Adenoma _____

3. Aneursym _____

4. Arteriovenous _____

5. Arteriovenous malformation (AVM) _____

6. Astrocytes _____

7. Bone flap _____

8. Central nervous system (CNS) _____

9. Embolization _____

10. Intracranial pressure (ICP) _____

11. Stereotactic _____

Label the following diagram of a neuron.

12. _____

13. _____

14. _____

15. _____

16. _____

17. _____

18. _____

19. _____

20. _____

21. _____

22. _____

23. _____

24. _____

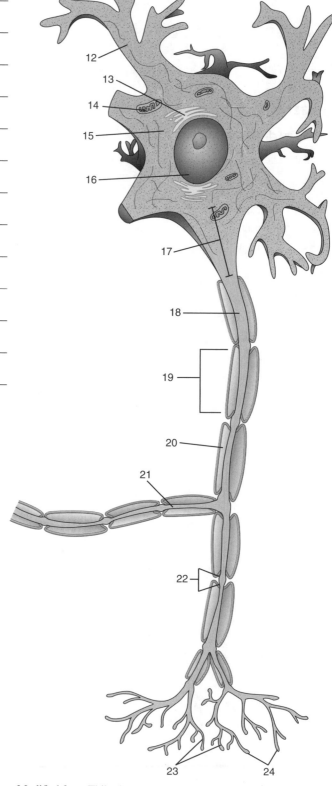

Modified from Thibodeau G, Patton K: *Anatomy and physiology,*
ed 6, St Louis, 2007, Mosby.

Provide a short answer for each question or statement.

25. The brain is divided into three main sections; what are they?

    a. _____

    b. _____

    c. _____

26. Describe the three protective coverings of the brain.

    a. _____

    b. _____

    c. _____

27. What are the common signs and symptoms of carpal tunnel syndrome? _____

    _____

    _____

    _____

    _____

28. Why are implanted dorsal column stimulators used and what do they do? _____

    _____

    _____

29. Why would your patient undergo a rhizotomy? _____

    _____

30. What is a disk herniation and why does it occur? _____

    _____

    _____

    _____

31. What must a surgical tech do to ensure the patient's safety during the postoperative phase after a halo brace has

been applied? _____

_____

_____

32. What are the possible complications after a procedure of the spine? _____

_____

_____

33. What procedure is performed to remove a tumor from the vestibular branch of the eighth cranial nerve?

_____

34. What is the difference between craniectomy and craniotomy? _____

_____

_____

35. What is CJD? _____

36. What are common diagnostic procedures that might be performed during the perioperative phase?

_____

_____

_____

_____

_____

_____

SEQUENCING

Number the following steps of stereotactic surgery in the correct sequence.

37. _____ The patient returns to the operating room, and the coordinates are loaded into the system's computer.

38. _____ A stereotactic head frame is attached to the patient's head with skull pins.

39. _____ The frame is removed.

40. _____ The patient undergoes an MRI or a CT scan to locate the target and determine the coordinates.

41. _____ The incisions are closed.

42. _____ Instrumentation is introduced through the burr hole as needed for the procedure.

43. _____ A burr hole is placed.

296

MATCHING

Match each term with the correct definition.

44. _____ Narrow path that leads directly into the fourth ventricle

45. _____ Outer tissue layer of the cerebrum

46. _____ Continuous connection between the spinal cord and the pons

47. _____ Layer of meninges that is closest to the brain

48. _____ Ligament that connects one spinous process of a vertebra to another vertebra

49. _____ Small bulges that occur throughout the surface of the cerebrum

50. _____ Large, deep furrows in the cerebrum

51. _____ Protective housing of the brain

a. Skull
b. Cerebral aqueduct
c. Medulla oblongata
d. Cerebral cortex
e. Cerebral peduncles
f. Gyri
g. Fissures
h. Ligamentum flavum
i. Pia mater
j. Dura mater

TRUE/FALSE

Indicate whether the statement is true or false.

52. Whenever the brain is manipulated surgically, the possibility of postoperative seizures arises.

_____ True   _____ False

53. The most common type of external stabilization of the cervical spine is the halo brace.

_____ True   _____ False

54. The patient is positioned for back surgery before induction and intubation.

_____ True   _____ False

55. The cranium is a closed cavity, and any pressure from excess fluid, such as blood, can impinge on brain tissue, causing injury and permanent damage.

_____ True   _____ False

56. Brain tissue does not have sensory nerves, and procedures can be performed under local anesthesia with monitored sedation.

_____ True   _____ False

57. A bone flap is created in the cranium by drilling burr holes and making cuts in the bone between the holes.

_____ True   _____ False

58. The procedure in which burr holes are drilled into the cranium to release intracranial pressure is called a craniotomy.

_____ True   _____ False

59. The autonomic nervous system is a voluntary system that transmits signals for vital functions such as the heart rate, respiration, and digestion.

_____ True   _____ False

60. The body has 8 cervical vertebrae, 12 thoracic vertebrae, 4 lumbar vertebrae, and 5 sacral vertebrae.

_____ True   _____ False

61. The surgical goal of ulnar nerve transposition is to free the ulnar nerve from a groove on the medial epicondyle.

_____ True   _____ False

62. Percutaneous cordotomy may be performed as a minimally invasive technique.

_____ True   _____ False

63. Aneurysm clips are supplied as permanent devices.

_____ True   _____ False

64. AVM is an abnormal communication between the cerebral arteries and veins.

_____ True   _____ False

65. DBS has been used to treat movement disorders, such as Parkinson's disease, and some pain disorders.

_____ True   _____ False

MULTIPLE CHOICE

Choose the most correct answer to complete the question or statement.

66. Which of the following procedures begins with the removal of a fat graft from the abdomen?
    a. Lumbar laminectomy
    b. Craniotomy
    c. Transsphenoidal hypophysectomy
    d. Nerve transposition

67. Removal of a diseased _____ is performed when the disk impinges on nerves, causing pain and dysfunction.
    a. Intervertebral disk
    b. Lamina
    c. Ventricle
    d. Meninge

68. Stabilization of the spinal column may be achieved with _____.
    a. Bone grafts
    b. Plates
    c. Rods
    d. All of the above

69. Procedures of the pituitary require techniques and instruments across two specialties: neurosurgery and _____ surgery.
    a. Orthopedic
    b. Nasal
    c. Dental
    d. Vascular

70. Which of the following are considered specialty sponges used in neurosurgery? (Select all that apply.)
    a. Cotton balls
    b. Cervical pledgets
    c. Neuro patties
    d. 2 × 2s

71. There are _____ pairs of spinal nerves.
    a. 15
    b. 31
    c. 36
    d. 40

72. The vertebral column is composed of
_____ bones, or vertebrae.
   a. 22
   b. 30
   c. 33
   d. 35

73. During a nerve repair, which of the following
sutures would be appropriate for the anastomosis?
   a. 3-0 or 4-0 Prolene
   b. 6-0 or 7-0 nylon
   c. 4-0 silk
   d. 6-0 chromic

74. In which of the following procedures would a
Penrose drain be used as a retractor?
   a. Ulnar nerve transposition
   b. Lumbar laminectomy
   c. Spinal fixation
   d. Carpal tunnel release

75. Which of the following incisions would be
appropriate for carpal tunnel release?
   a. Midline lumbar incision
   b. Long incision over the lateral elbow
   c. Curvilinear or longitudinal incision in the palm
      that extends to the wrist
   d. Paramedian

76. During spinal surgery for tumor removal,
_____ may be used to restore continuity
of the dura.
   a. Portion of the patient's pericranium
   b. Bovine pericardium
   c. Biosynthetic dura substitutes
   d. All of the above

77. Lumbar laminectomy is performed to access the
lumbar spinal cord and remove a portion of the
_____.
   a. Lumbar disk
   b. Lumbar lamina
   c. Intervertebral disk
   d. Ligamentum flavum

78. The surgeon begins a laminectomy with a
_____ to remove the spinous process.
   a. Leksell rongeur
   b. Addison rongeur
   c. Cobb elevator
   d. Midas Rex

79. _____ is performed to improve blood
flow to an ischemic area of the brain.
   a. AV shunt
   b. Cerebral revascularization
   c. Burr holes
   d. Endoscopic ventriculoscopy

80. Longer term complications of a craniotomy include
all of the following except:
   a. Infection of the bone flap or brain tissue
   b. Persistent seizure activity
   c. Unresolved neurological deficits
   d. Aneurysm formation

81. Common types of headrests used in neurosurgery
include all of the following except:
   a. Light-Veley
   b. Mayfield
   c. Three-pin fixation
   d. Gardner-Wells

82. The patient may be positioned in the sitting position
or prone on chest rolls or a laminectomy frame for
which procedure?
   a. Lumbar laminectomy
   b. Lumbar rhizotomy
   c. Posterior cervical laminectomy
   d. Ulnar nerve transposition

CASE STUDIES

Case Study 1

Read the following case study and answer the questions.

Your patient has been recently diagnosed with an endocrine-dependent malignant
tumor of the pituitary gland.

83. What signs or symptoms did your patient most likely have when she arrived at the

physician's office? _____

_____

299

84. What procedure will the surgeon suggest to the patient as a potential cure?

_____

85. How will the surgeon describe to the patient the potential postoperative complications

for this procedure? _____

_____

86. Where will the incision be? _____

Case Study 2

Your surgical case today is an open craniotomy for removal of a tumor. The surgeon is going to "turn a flap," including the bone.

87. As the scrub, what is your responsibility with regard to the bone if it is removed from

the patient? _____

_____

INTERNET EXERCISES

Internet Exercise 1

*Using your favorite search engine, type in the keywords **cerebral aneurysm.** After you get to a research area, answer the following questions about your findings.*

88. Are there different types of aneurysm? _____

88. If so, name several types. _____

_____

89. Did you find any information on the cause or causes of an aneurysm? _____

_____

91. In the following space, draw the type or types of aneurysm that you found and label it/them.

Internet Exercise 2

Using your favorite search engine, look for medical mnemonics. When you find a site, give the Web page and then list the mnemonics that describe neuroanatomy or neuropathology that you think will help you with this unit.

92. Web page: _____

Mnemonics: _____

_____

_____

300